WELL
WOMAN

Dr. Miriam Stoppard

WELL WOMAN

HEALTHCARE

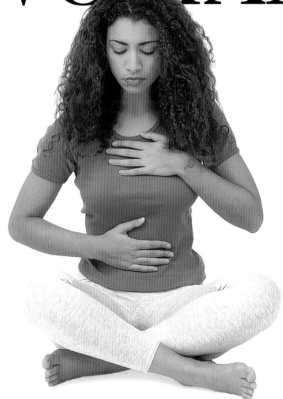

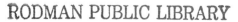
DK PUBLISHING, INC.

A D   JAN   1999

DE:

SENIOR MANAGING
ART EDITOR   Lynne Brown

MANAGING EDITOR   Jemima Dunne

SENIOR ART EDITOR   Karen Ward

SENIOR EDITORS   Nicky Adamson,
Penny Warren

US EDITOR   Jill Hamilton

US CONSULTANT   Elsa-Grace Giardina, MD

PRODUCTION   Antony Heller

First American Edition, 1998
2 4 6 8 10 9 7 5 3 1
Published in the United States by
DK Publishing Inc., 95 Madison Avenue,
New York, New York 10016

Visit us on the World Wide Web at
http://www.dk.com

Library of Congress Cataloging-in-Publication Data

Stoppard, Miriam.
Well woman / Miriam Stoppard. -- 1st American
ed. p. cm. -- (DK healthcare series)
Includes index.
ISBN 0-7894-3091-6
1. Gynecology--Popular works. 2. Women--
Health and hygiene. I. Title. II. Series.
RG121.S863 1998
618.1--dc21   97-43771
                                        CIP

Reproduced by Colourscan, Singapore and
IGS, Radstock, Avon
Printed in Hong Kong by Wing King Tong

CONTENTS

INTRODUCTION 6

CHAPTER 1

HEALTHY FEMALE BODY 7

THE FEMALE BODY 8
MENSTRUATION 10
FERTILITY AND CONCEPTION 12
CONTRACEPTION 14
MENOPAUSE 18

CHAPTER 2

GENITAL PROBLEMS 21

PRURITIS VULVAE 22
VAGINAL DISCHARGE 23
THRUSH 24
TRICHOMONIASIS 25
CERVICAL CANCER 26
CYSTITIS 28
PROLAPSE 30
INCONTINENCE 32

CHAPTER 3

MENSTRUAL PROBLEMS 33

PREMENSTRUAL SYNDROME 34
AMENORRHEA 35
ABNORMAL BLEEDING 36
DYSMENORRHEA 37
MENORRHAGIA 38

CHAPTER 4

PELVIC PROBLEMS 39

ENDOMETRIOSIS 40
FIBROIDS 41
OVARIAN CYSTS 42
OVARIAN CANCER 44
UTERINE CANCER 45
PELVIC INFLAMMATORY DISEASE 46

CHAPTER 5

SEXUAL PROBLEMS 47

PAINFUL INTERCOURSE 48
LACK OF SEX DRIVE 49
VAGINISMUS 50

CHAPTER 6

SEXUALLY TRANSMITTED DISEASES 51

GENITAL HERPES 52
GENITAL WARTS 53
CHLAMYDIA 54
GONORRHEA 55
SYPHILIS 56
HIV/AIDS 57

CHAPTER 7

FERTILITY PROBLEMS 59

· PROBLEMS WITH FERTILITY 60
MISCARRIAGE 66
ECTOPIC PREGNANCY 68

CHAPTER 8

INVESTIGATIONS AND OPERATIONS 69

PELVIC EXAMINATION • CERVICAL SMEAR
• COLPOSCOPY • ENDOMETRIAL BIOPSY
• HYSTEROSCOPY • ULTRASOUND SCAN
• HYSTEROSALPINGOGRAM • LAPAROSCOPY
• MYOMECTOMY • HYSTERECTOMY
• CONE BIOPSY/LLETZ • D&C/ERPC
ST
• TER

INTRODUCTION

ALTHOUGH MANY MEDICAL conditions affect both men and women, there are aspects of women's health that are unique to them. As a result of the complicated chemistry of the female hormones and the position of the reproductive organs deep within the abdomen, many women may experience some imbalance or health complication in this area at some point in their lives.

The good news is that medical research has dramatically improved our understanding of how women's bodies work, and how problems can be prevented or eliminated at an early stage. Understanding the function of hormones has enabled scientists to develop medicines that can often avoid the more invasive treatments that were a necessity in the past. Screening, diagnostic tests, and microsurgery are used to detect potential medical conditions early on, providing reassurance or prompt treatment.

In the excitement of rapid scientific advances, there was a tendency for doctors sometimes to overwhelm women with their superior knowledge, leaving their patients feeling bewildered and no longer in control. Today, however, it is widely recognized that women have the right to know what is happening to them, what is possible and what is not, and why certain treatments are recommended and what they involve. This book is designed to lead you through conditions and diseases that particularly affect women, and the procedures likely to be used to diagnose and treat them.

Maintaining health – being a well woman – means being aware when something is amiss, taking advantage of screening, and being informed – so that if you need treatment, you can have confidence in what is being offered by your doctor, and what it means for your future.

CHAPTER 1

HEALTHY FEMALE BODY

The female human body has adapted over
millions of years to perform its biological functions
efficiently. In this chapter, the major physical
changes we undergo as we grow older are explored
in detail, beginning with menstruation, leading
on to fertility and conception, and finally to
menopause. These changes are explained together
with various ways of dealing with them. Knowledge
is power, and understanding what is happening to
you at these different stages in your life can help
you make informed decisions.

THE FEMALE BODY

We start being female from the moment of conception, when an X sperm fertilizes the female egg. After just a few weeks of development in the uterus, an embryo's female characteristics are clearly visible. Even at this early stage, the female genitals – the labia, clitoris, vagina, and primitive uterus – are all present, and the ovaries already contain a supply of eggs, many more than are shed monthly from puberty to menopause.

THE BEGINNING OF FERTILITY

At puberty, the potent female hormones, estrogen and progesterone, begin to create a cycle of fertility. Every month the ovaries

MILESTONES IN DEVELOPMENT

From babyhood, the differences in body shape between boys and girls are noticeable. Girls tend to have more rounded buttocks and their angled thigh bones are another obvious difference. At about nine or ten the pelvic bones begin to grow, and more fat is deposited on the thighs, hips, and breasts. By 12, nipples have budded and pubic hair sprouts. By about 18, bone growth is completed and adult height is reached.
The next time of change is the period known as the climacteric, between the onset and ending of menopause symptoms. At menopause, the ovaries run out of eggs, estrogen and progesterone hormones stop being released, and menstrual periods cease.

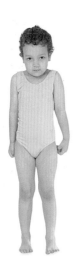

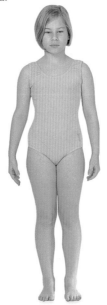

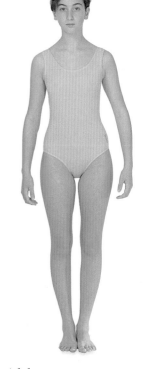

Young child
Even from a very young age, a girl's body is more rounded than a boy's.

Prepubertal
From 9–10, girls start to grow rapidly and their pelvic bones become more developed.

Adolescent
At 14, most girls are sexually mature, but they have not yet reached adult height.

release an egg, which travels down one of the two fallopian tubes that connect the ovaries with the uterus. If the egg is not fertilized, it is eventually expelled from the body during menstruation.

This very complicated combination of hormones and biology developed solely to enable us to become pregnant and give birth, thus ensuring the continuation of our species. If the egg *is* fertilized by sperm, pregnancy results.

Pregnancy and Birth

Pregnancy is divided into three distinct stages, called trimesters, each one lasting about three months. During the first, your body starts to make the adjustments that will enable you to carry the baby to term: your heart and breathing rates increase, the uterus thickens and grows, and the size and weight of your breasts increase. During the second and third trimesters, nipples enlarge and darken, the heart works twice as hard as that of a nonpregnant woman, and the uterus continues to expand outward to accommodate the fetus; during the last few weeks of pregnancy, walking becomes uncomfortable and hands and feet may swell.

On or about the 40th week of pregnancy, you will go into labor and give birth, an event like no other you will ever experience. No one knows precisely how labor starts, but there is increasing evidence to show that the baby plays a major role. The onset of labor is triggered by the secretion of hormones, one of which is produced by the baby. The uterus responds by starting to contract regularly at shorter and shorter intervals and with increasing force until the baby is expelled from the womb.

Within about six weeks of the birth of the baby, the uterus should have shrunk back to its normal prepregnancy size – from about 2lb (1kg) at the end of the pregnancy to about 2oz (50g) – and within several weeks after that, menstruation will usually recommence. The cycle of fertility has begun all over again.

Limiting Fertility

We are fertile for well over 30 years and are theoretically capable of many pregnancies. Much ingenuity, therefore, has gone into evolving ways to limit the effects of such fertility. Until this century, however, methods were hit or miss, depending on a mixture of avoidance of sex at what was believed to be the "crucial" time of the month (the calendar method), or on the man withdrawing before ejaculating (coitus interruptus).

Today, we have the ability to manipulate our fertility much more accurately through various artificial methods of contraception, including oral contraceptives and intrauterine or barrier devices (see p. 14). For both men and women, this ability has probably been one of the most significant developments in history: it has allowed us to control the size of our families; for us as women, it has also meant freedom to decide not just when, but if, we wish to become mothers.

The End of Fertility

The great milestone of middle age is menopause. In the years leading up to it, our body prepares us for the end of fertility: periods can become irregular, sometimes heavy, and we may not ovulate every month.

Just as the beginning of menstruation brings about significant changes to our body, so does the end. The symptoms that signal the passing of our reproductive years include hot flushes, sweating, fragile bones, and dryness of the vagina; lowering estrogen levels can not only lead to a redistribution of body fat but also make us more susceptible to illnesses, such as heart disease and osteoporosis. But the advent of hormone replacement therapy (HRT) and other treatments, and a greater understanding of the importance of diet and exercise in maintaining health, has minimized such discomfort. What was once referred to ominously as *the* change of life can be demoted to being merely one of many changes in a busy and productive life.

MENSTRUATION

The medical term for the beginning of menstruation is menarche. The advent of menarche (usually about the age of 12 in developed countries) signals that a girl is entering her fertile life. Cyclical female hormone production starts and ovulation each month is a possibility, although few girls ovulate consistently in their first year or two of menstruation.

HORMONAL EFFECTS

Hormone production is not smooth in the beginning and may result in peaks and valleys, explaining why a teenage girl can become rebellious, moody, confused, and mixed up. It also leads to the maturing of a girl's body and the appearance of adult characteristics, such as breasts and pubic hair.

The regular production of female hormones results in various changes in our bodies throughout the month. In the first half of the cycle, estrogen is produced, which makes the skin bloom and raises our mood so that we feel that we can tackle anything. It also affects the appearance of vaginal discharge prior to ovulation; at this time of the month it is thin, clear, and runny, with very little odor.

After ovulation, progesterone begins to show its effects. Vaginal secretions become thicker, opaque, more rubbery, and definitely have a fishy odor. The breasts enlarge, become heavy and tender, and toward menstruation the nipples may tingle and feel sore. This is perfectly normal and the effects subside on or before the beginning of bleeding. Progesterone can cause acne-like spots on the face at this time of the month, and very few of us escape without having one or two of these at some point in our lives. They should disappear when the menstrual period starts.

MENSTRUAL PROBLEMS

Most of the time, monthly periods follow a predictable pattern. For most women some of the time, however, problems can and do occur, particularly during the early years of menstruation and in the premenopausal years, as the body prepares itself for menstruation to cease. Disorders can range from **premenstrual syndrome** (which about 75 percent of us suffer from at one time or another in our lives) to painful periods (**dysmenorrhea**). Common menstrual problems are described in chapter 3.

THE REPRODUCTIVE ORGANS

The reproductive glands in women are the two ovaries. From puberty they release the ova (eggs), and manufacture the sex hormones, estrogen and progesterone. Estrogen influences the development of female body shape, enlargement of the breasts, and the menstrual cycle. Each month an egg is released by the ovaries and travels down one of the two fallopian tubes to the uterus, a hollow structure in the center of the pelvis; if the egg is not fertilized, menstruation occurs.

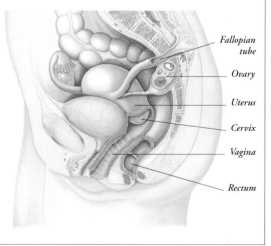

Fallopian tube

Ovary

Uterus

Cervix

Vagina

Rectum

THE MENSTRUAL CYCLE

The average cycle is about 28 days, but a cycle can be as long as 33 or as short as 26 days. It is counted from the first day of bleeding to the last day before the next period.

Days 1–13
At the beginning of the cycle, levels of the female hormones – estrogen and progesterone – are low. Then the pituitary gland (which masterminds the production and distribution of hormones in the body) secretes follicle-stimulating hormone (FSH). This stimulates the ovary to grow egg follicles which, in their turn, secrete estrogen. Estrogen levels rise, encouraging the lining of the uterus (the endometrium) to thicken and prepare for a possible pregnancy.

Day 14 Ovulation
When estrogen levels peak, this stimulates production of yet more FSH as well as luteinizing hormone (LH). This hormone causes the follicle to burst, releasing the ripe egg. This is ovulation.

Days 15–28
The egg starts to move down the fallopian tube and the follicle matures into a corpus luteum (small mass of yellow tissue), which secretes large amounts of progesterone in the second half of the month. Three days prior to menstruation, the corpus luteum begins to age, and progesterone levels fall. If unfertilized, the egg is expelled and the endometrium is shed. Menstruation has begun.

MENSTRUAL HYGIENE

Menstruation is no longer the taboo subject it once was. When I was young, it was said that young girls shouldn't wash their hair or bathe during menstruation because the blood might go to the brain. This is nonsense, and the general rule should be to bathe as often as you want to, or at least shower or spongebathe, so that you feel comfortable. Wash yourself with ordinary soap and water.

For protection, some girls prefer to use sanitary napkins and these are ideal to begin with, but you might also want to consider tampons, which can be more comfortable, hygienic, and discreet. One good way to experiment with tampons is to try them at the same time as a friend. I remember doing so with one of my college friends as we stood in adjacent toilets and gave running commentaries to each other on our progress. If you do use tampons, don't forget about them; they should be changed every four to six hours.

MENSTRUATION AND SEX

To protect yourself from sexually transmitted diseases, it is best to use a condom when having intercourse with any new partner, but it is even more important during menstruation. This is because blood-borne viruses such as HIV, hepatitis B, and hepatitis C are transmitted more easily by unprotected sex during menstruation than at any other time of the month.

SEE ALSO:
Dysmenorrhea, *page 37*
Menstrual Problems, *page 33*
Premenstrual Syndrome, *page 34*
Vaginal Discharge, *page 23*

FERTILITY AND CONCEPTION

Fertility is the term generally used to describe the ability to have a baby; conception is the first step to pregnancy.

During sexual intercourse, millions of sperm are released into the vagina. At ovulation, an egg is released from the ovary and begins to travel down the fallopian tube toward the uterus. The mucus at the cervix becomes thinner to enable sperm to travel up through the cervix and uterus toward the egg. Only an extremely small proportion of the sperm originally ejaculated reaches the fallopian tubes. These sperm cluster around the egg until one actually penetrates its outer shell, when fertilization takes place. The rest then drop off and die.

Conception is the implantation of the fertilized egg in the uterus. The ovaries increase their levels of female hormones to prepare the lining of the uterus to support the pregnancy until the placenta can take over. It is this increased level of hormone production that can cause early symptoms of pregnancy such as morning sickness, giddiness, fainting, tingling in the breasts, and a desire to urinate frequently. If conception does not occur, hormone production diminishes, thus triggering the monthly menstrual period.

GAUGING FERTILITY

A woman's fertility depends on several events, but the most crucial point to remember is that even someone who ovulates regularly is fertile for only about three days each month.

A woman's age is a significant factor in determining her fertility: she reaches her peak at about the age of 24 (in fact, at exactly the same age as a man reaches his peak). Eggs decline in quality with increasing age. There is a definite decline after about the age of 30 and it is very rare, although not impossible, for a woman to conceive after the age of about 50. Even with normal fertilization, however, the uterine environment during the premeno- pausal years may be much less favorable and the egg will therefore have much less chance of survival.

THE TIMING OF INTERCOURSE

To ensure fertilization, intercourse must occur within a day or so of ovulation – you can confirm that ovulation has taken place with an ovulation kit, or by checking your vaginal discharge (see p. 23).

Sperm can survive within a woman's body for between two and three days after intercourse takes place; an egg is viable for only about two days following ovulation. During an average 28-day cycle, therefore, the fertile period is comparatively short. Although every woman's pattern is slightly different, you are more likely to conceive in the middle of your menstrual cycle and less likely to conceive very early in the menstrual cycle or within the last few days before your next menstrual period.

HOW GENES DETERMINE SEX

Each ovum (egg) and each sperm consists of 23 chromosomes; 22 of these pair with each other and on fertilization make up the genetic material of the future child. The 23rd chromosome determines a child's sex, and is X (female) or Y (male). The father produces X and Y sperm, while a woman's eggs are always X. If an X sperm unites with the egg, the child will be female; if a Y sperm unites with it, the child will be male.

The other chromosomes contain genetic material that determine such characteristics as hair and eye color, as well as the tendency to inherit certain diseases, such as cystic fibrosis, and conditions such as color blindness.

BEGINNING OF LIFE

Cell division

Once the egg is fertilized, it quickly divides, first into two cells, then four, then eight, and so on. These early cells are called totipotential cells because they could develop into any part of the body.

TWO CELLS   FOUR CELLS   EIGHT CELLS   BLASTOCYST

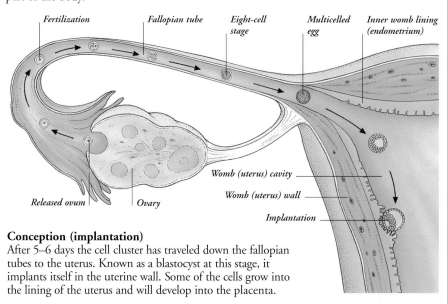

Fertilization   *Fallopian tube*   *Eight-cell stage*   *Multicelled egg*   *Inner womb lining (endometrium)*

Womb (uterus) cavity

Womb (uterus) wall

Implantation

Released ovum   *Ovary*

Conception (implantation)

After 5–6 days the cell cluster has traveled down the fallopian tubes to the uterus. Known as a blastocyst at this stage, it implants itself in the uterine wall. Some of the cells grow into the lining of the uterus and will develop into the placenta.

If you menstruate regularly, there are ways to confirm when you ovulate. The easiest way is the temperature method and by examining your cervical mucus. In the temperature method, take your temperature first thing in the morning throughout the month; when it stays up 0.4°F (0.2°C) three days in a row, and there is no other possible cause, this usually indicates ovulation. With the mucus method, you should examine your mucus regularly throughout the cycle: it should become slippery and clear, and you should feel "wet," two or three days prior to ovulation. An ovulation kit available from pharmacies is the most accurate method.

It isn't true that conception is more likely if you have intercourse very frequently; in fact, the opposite may be true – the more often a man ejaculates, the fewer sperm are contained in his ejaculate each time. If you are anxious to become pregnant, therefore, it may be a good idea to abstain from sex for a few days prior to ovulation to build up the numbers of sperm, or at least to confine it to alternate days.

SEE ALSO:

Fertility Problems, *page 59*
Menopause, *page 18*
Menstrual Problems, *page 33*
Menstruation, *page 10*

CONTRACEPTION

If you need your contraceptive method to be nearly 100 percent effective without resorting to sterilization, there are two choices. You can use the combined contraceptive pill or the progesterone intrauterine device, which prevents conception and the implantation of the fertilized egg.

The next most effective means is what is called the "mini-pill" (progesterone-only pill) and the IUD (intrauterine device), followed by the various barrier methods.

WHAT METHOD IS BEST FOR ME?

The best method for you is the one that is most effective, but effectiveness can be judged by two criteria: theoretical and actual. Invariably, the latter has a higher failure rate because of the human element.

The least effective, largely because of human error, are the so-called "natural" methods, the ones that rely on determining safe periods and abstaining from intercourse during that time. Since the medical complications of pregnancy outweigh those of the combined pill, getting pregnant is always more risky than taking the pill. Contraceptives with the greatest risk are those with the highest failure rate.

Your choice of birth control will probably change during your fertile years. No one method is ideal for this length of time, punctuated as it may be by planned pregnancies and changes in sexual partners. You need to think about all the forms of contraception and match them to your personality, sexual habits, and stage in life.

NATURAL METHODS

These methods include the oldest forms of contraception and consist of periodic abstinence, breast-feeding, and withdrawal.

PERIODIC ABSTINENCE

Abstaining from intercourse during the time of ovulation is based on calculations using the calendar, plus the rise and fall of the woman's body temperature and the appearance of vaginal secretions. Using these indicators, you can decide to abstain from penetrative sex during ovulation.

A home ovulation test kit is the best method of detecting ovulation but there are older methods. The first is the calendar or rhythm method, which requires you to chart your cycle and abstain from intercourse during your fertile days.

The symptothermal method involves taking your temperature and observing the consistency and color of your vaginal secretions. By taking your temperature with a very accurate thermometer at the same time every day (preferably first thing in the morning), you should be able to notice a rise of a fraction of a degree during the second half of your cycle, providing you are not suffering from an infection.

The second part of the routine is known as the Billings method. Your vaginal secretions also change during your cycle. Immediately after menstruation, you will be comparatively dry. Then, as the mucus builds up, you may notice it becoming thick, cloudy, and sticky. This changes to clear, stretchy, and abundant at the time of ovulation, when you should avoid intercourse.

WHAT ARE THE RISKS?

These methods are hopeless for women with irregular cycles and have a high failure rate. They require a strong commitment from both partners. Although there are no risks to health, there may be to relationships and, with a comparatively high failure rate, problems of unwanted pregnancy. You need at least six months to establish these techniques properly and determine what is normal for you.

BREAST-FEEDING

Breast-feeding over a 24-hour time period changes the levels of hormones and prevents ovulation. However, it is not a

BARRIER DEVICES

Condoms

Condoms are plastic sheaths that create a physical barrier to prevent sperm from reaching the ovum. They must be used with spermicides as well.

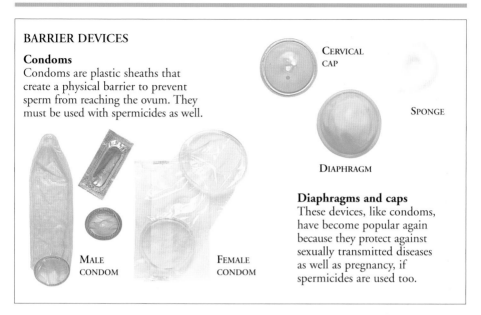

CERVICAL CAP

SPONGE

DIAPHRAGM

MALE CONDOM

FEMALE CONDOM

Diaphragms and caps

These devices, like condoms, have become popular again because they protect against sexually transmitted diseases as well as pregnancy, if spermicides are used too.

---

reliable means of birth control and becomes particularly unreliable once the 24-hour feeding regime is reduced. Just because you don't have a period during breast-feeding does not mean that you are not producing eggs and you must make sure, therefore, that you use some form of contraception, such as the mini-pill.

WITHDRAWAL

This is another ancient method with a very high failure rate, where the penis is withdrawn just before ejaculation. It doesn't require discussion about methods with doctors and at clinics and requires no financial outlay, but it also leaves much of the responsibility with the man.

BARRIER METHODS

These methods physically block the sperm from reaching the ovum or they chemically inactivate them.

MALE CONDOM

The condom is a latex rubber or plastic sheath that is placed over the erect penis before penetration. It should be lubricated and emptied of air so that it doesn't burst inside the vagina. It works by preventing the sperm from entering the vagina.

The condom has been available for many years, and can be bought in a variety of retail outlets. It is widely used even by those who use another form of contraception because of the danger of sexually transmitted diseases, especially AIDS. I would therefore advise all women who have not been engaged in monogamous relationships for at least five years to insist on using male or female condoms.

FEMALE CONDOM

The female condom is designed to line the inside of the vagina. It consists of a lubricated plastic sheath with an anchoring ring to keep it in place within the vagina and an outer ring that holds the sheath open to allow insertion of the penis.

It allows a woman to control the method of contraception as well as providing good protection against sexually transmitted diseases, but has the disadvantage of being slightly awkward to insert. It is as effective as the male condom in preventing pregnancy.

CONTRACEPTION: CONTINUED

DIAPHRAGM AND CERVICAL CAP

The diaphragm, a dome of rubber with a coiled metal spring in its rim, is made in different sizes, depending on a woman's internal shape and size. It fits diagonally across the vagina and is used with a spermicidal agent; it must be left in place for six hours after intercourse.

The cervical cap is smaller and more rigid and fits over the cervix, where it is held in place by suction. Like the diaphragm, it must be fitted to size and used in conjunction with a spermicide. The diaphragm and cap work by preventing sperm from reaching the cervix. They must be refitted regularly, because of childbirth or weight gain or loss.

CONTRACEPTIVE SPONGE

This is an old form of contraception now updated with contemporary materials. These days it is usually made of polyurethane foam and is impregnated with spermicide. The sponge is moistened with water to activate the spermicide and left in place for six hours after intercourse.

SPERMICIDES

The use of a spermicide is essential with these barrier methods to ensure their effectiveness. Spermicides are not effective on their own since they must be at the cervix, not just somewhere in the vagina. They come in many forms, including aerosols, pessaries, foams, gels, and creams. Some need to be inserted 15 minutes before intercourse, and a spermicide should not be washed away for at least six hours afterward. Spermicides seem to provide added protection against contracting sexually transmitted diseases.

HORMONAL METHODS

These methods use hormones to suppress ovulation. They interfere with the cervical mucus, making it thick and impenetrable to sperm, and thin the uterine lining so that conception cannot occur. Forms include the combined pill, the low-dose mini-pill, hormonal injections, and implants. The postcoital pill also contains hormones.

The *combined pill* uses synthetic progestogen and estrogen to suppress ovulation. It must be taken for the full course of either 21 or 28 days to be effective. The *low-dose mini-pill* contains progestogen only. It is slightly less reliable because ovulation may occur. Estrogen is implicated in some of the side-effects of the combined pill because of its effect on the circulatory system.

Injectable contraceptives contain only progestogens and are administered every two or three months. They are ideal for women who have difficulty remembering to take the pill regularly. *Implants* are also available, usually inserted under the skin of the upper arm, remaining active for five years. Both of these methods are relatively free from side-effects. The return to fertility can sometimes be slow after an injectable contraceptive, but is usually quite soon after an implant is removed. There may be some breakthrough bleeding.

HORMONAL CONTRACEPTION

Advantages
- The most effective method
- Regulates menstruation and reduces pain and bleeding
- Reduces the effects of PMS
- Reduces the incidence of benign cysts and ovarian cancers, and protects against brittle bones (osteoporosis)

Disadvantages
- Slightly increased risk of thrombosis in women using this method
- Occasional breakthrough bleeding with some forms
- It requires motivation to take the mini-pill at the same time every day

POSTCOITAL METHODS

There are two means of preventing conception after unprotected sex and they must be started within 1–5 days after intercourse, but they are not recommended as a routine form of birth control.

The hormonal method involves a short high-dose course of the combined pill. It is not entirely clear how this method works in preventing pregnancy. For women who cannot take the high-dose pill, a copper-bearing IUD can be inserted within five days of unprotected intercourse; this prevents a possible pregnancy.

WHAT ARE THE RISKS?

A pill containing estrogen may not be suitable for you if you are overweight; if you smoke; are over 35; suffer from diabetes, high blood pressure, a heart condition, deep-vein thrombosis, or migraine.

INTRAUTERINE DEVICE

This is a plastic or copper-containing device inserted into the uterus and left there. It probably works by causing an inflammation in the uterus that kills the sperm, or by preventing the fertilized egg

INTRAUTERINE DEVICES

Advantages
• One of the most reliable methods (second only to hormonal contraception)
• No need to take pills every day
• Do not interfere with ovulation or breast-feeding

Disadvantages
• Can be expelled without the user being aware of it
• Copper-containing devices are known to cause occasional complications in some women
• May increase pain and bleeding during menstruation

from implanting in the uterine lining. An IUD is immediately effective in preventing pregnancy and does not interfere with breast-feeding or your natural hormonal balance. There are many different shapes and sizes of IUDs. Most have a tail for easy removal and as a quick check that they are still in place.

PROGESTERONE INTRAUTERINE DEVICE

The progesterone IUD is similar to other IUDs in that it sits in the uterus. However, because it contains a progesterone hormone it actively prevents the lining of the uterus from increasing in thickness and causes the mucus in the cervix to remain thick. It also acts as a physical barrier to conception by being present in the uterus. In some women it suppresses ovulation. Overall, it is a very good contraceptive, lasting for a minimum of three years.

RISKS AND DISADVANTAGES

IUDs are not suitable for young women who have not had children. These devices have been implicated in cases of perforation of the uterus, septic abortion, **pelvic inflammatory disease**, and **ectopic pregnancy**. They may increase bleeding and pain during menstruation, so they are not suitable for women with heavy periods. Expulsion of the devices is not uncommon and they are painful to insert in some cases.

Disadvantages of the progesterone IUD include possible risk of **ovarian cysts** and a shorter lifespan than some of the other copper-containing IUDs.

SEE ALSO:
Ectopic Pregnancy, *page 68*
Fertility and Conception, *page 12*
Menstruation, *page 10*
Ovarian Cysts, *page 42*
Pelvic Inflammatory Disease, *page 46*

MENOPAUSE

Strictly speaking, menopause is your last menstrual period, but you only become aware of this in retrospect, when you haven't had a period for a year. The average age of menopause in this country is 52, although it is not unusual to experience it during your early 40s or mid-50s.

STAGES OF MENOPAUSE

Menopause is also sometimes called the "climacteric." It encompasses three distinct stages: *premenopause,* the beginning of the climacteric (usually the early 40s) when periods may become heavy or irregular; *perimenopause,* the stage (usually a few years) on either side of your last period when physical symptoms such as hot flushes begin and periods become more irregular; and *postmenopause,* which encompasses the rest of your life, after your periods stop.

CAN I PREDICT MY MENOPAUSE?

Most menstrual periods stop gradually. A few years before menopause, they may become irregular: you have them for several months then skip a month or two, then start again, with the interval between becoming longer and longer until eventually they stop completely. If you are over 50 and have not had a period for over six months, you have probably reached menopause.

There is no way that you can predict when your last period will be. The age at which you first menstruated could be significant, and the earlier you start, the later you finish. The age at which your mother experienced menopause may also affect when you have yours, although this is difficult to prove. Whether you took the oral contraceptive pill and the age at which you had your first and last child do *not* affect the timing.

It seems most likely that each one of us has our own built-in biological clock that dictates both when we start to menstruate and when we stop, although a variety of physical factors including diet, smoking, and obesity can either slow the clock down or speed it up.

PREMATURE MENOPAUSE

A premature natural menopause, which occurs before the age of 35, is very rare, affecting less than one percent of women.

Surgical removal of the ovaries (oophorectomy) is the most common cause of premature menopause and is carried out for a variety of reasons, such as a ruptured **ectopic pregnancy** or **ovarian cancer**. It is usually done as part of a total **hysterectomy**, which entails removal of both the ovaries, the fallopian tubes, and the uterus. Other factors that can cause an artificial menopause include radiation therapy (for stomach and pelvic cancers and, rarely, mumps).

For natural menopause, hormone replacement therapy is given immediately to offset possible problems arising from the earlier-than-usual loss of estrogen. Estrogen replacement therapy is used if the uterus has been removed.

LATE MENOPAUSE

Anyone still menstruating after the age of 55 is considered to have a late menopause. Late menopause can have health consequences, too, since your body is exposed to estrogen for longer than normal, which, theoretically, carries a slightly increased risk of uterine and breast cancer. You can protect yourself against this risk by making sure that you receive regular mammograms and pelvic examinations.

WHAT HAPPENS DURING THE CLIMACTERIC?

Many women experience the symptoms of estrogen deficiency during the time that menstruation begins to decline. Periods become less and less frequent and then menstruation finally stops. Old-fashioned phrases like the "change of life" imply that

SYMPTOMS

Nonphysical symptoms include:
- *Depression*
- *Irritability*
- *Tearfulness and inability to cope*
- *Loss of libido*
- *Insomnia*

Physical symptoms include:
- *Hot flushes*
- *Night sweats*
- *Itchiness of the perineum – vaginitis*
- *Pain during intercourse*
- *Fatigue and lack of energy*
- *Aches and pains as a result of softening bones*

menopause means an unavoidable decline in life. This is not so. In fact, most women find that life improves.

WHAT CAUSES MENOPAUSAL SYMPTOMS?

The decline in monthly menstrual periods is only a symptom of a parallel decline in the production of female hormones, particularly estrogen, by your body. What started at puberty with a first period and a change in your physical shape, now wanes as ovarian activity falls off and you fail to ovulate. Nearly all the symptoms of menopause may be attributed to these decreasing levels of estrogen in your blood.

SHOULD I SEE THE DOCTOR?

Three out of four menopausal women have symptoms that are worth treating and that should be treated. Don't grin and bear it. Decide to have the menopause you want, and seek medical advice and treatment. Don't ignore self-help remedies: there are many to try (see overleaf).

By far the most common menopausal symptoms are hot flushes, night sweats, and vaginal dryness; these can lead to other symptoms, such as insomnia and reduced sexual desire.

However, if any of the symptoms trouble you, make sure that you see your doctor immediately. It is never normal to have frequent heavy or painful periods nor to pass blood clots during menopause, so do consult your doctor if you experience any of these symptoms.

WHAT MIGHT THE DOCTOR DO?

By far the majority of women manage to cope with menopause reasonably easily. Because of the unsympathetic attitude of some male doctors, however, many women view it as something to be suffered and not worth treating. This is not so. Hormone replacement therapy can replace the estrogen deficiency so that the symptoms disappear. HRT is more than 90 percent effective. If you feel your doctor isn't being very helpful or sympathetic, or won't let you try hormone replacement therapy, go to another doctor.

HORMONE REPLACEMENT

Hormone replacement therapy (HRT) is the most effective way to relieve menopausal symptoms. It works essentially by replacing the hormones that the body loses: estrogen and progesterone.

HRT is available as tablets, patches, implants, and creams or pessaries. The first three are usually prescribed in a combined estrogen-progestogen (a synthetic form of progesterone) form, and all women who take them will have a monthly bleed when the progestogen phase of the course stops. Women who have had a total hysterectomy will be prescribed estrogen-only HRT.

Tablets are taken every day; skin patches need to be changed every three or four days; and implants, inserted by your doctor, need to be renewed every six months. Vaginal creams or pessaries only have a local effect and will not alleviate problems such as hot flushes and brittle bones.

MENOPAUSE: CONTINUED

With the end of the protective effects of female hormones, women are at equal risk with men from heart disease. Plenty of exercise and a low-fat diet with healthy combinations of foods will help to keep this problem at bay. Some emotional problems cannot be treated with hormone therapy alone and your doctor may prescribe tranquilizers and counseling to get you through the roughest patch.

ARE THERE NATURAL REMEDIES?

You don't always have to rely on medical doctors. Complementary therapies, such as homeopathy, aromatherapy, herbalism, yoga, and massage, all offer treatments for menopausal symptoms.

Homeopathic remedies
Many women consult homeopathic practitioners to relieve menopausal symptoms. Remedies – administered in minute doses – include *Lachesia* for hot flushes; *Pulsatilla* for insomnia, premenstrual syndrome, and joint pain; *Sepia* for dry vagina, thinning hair, and prolapse; *Sulfur* for itchy vulva and skin; *Bryonia* for PMS and breast pain; and *Belladonna* for night sweats.

Aromatherapy remedies
Essential oils from certain flowers and plants are also believed to relieve symptoms. Oils from cypress, geranium, and rose are recommended for heavy menstrual periods; avocado and wheatgerm for dry skin; juniper, lavender, and rosemary for muscle and joint pain; lavender and peppermint for headaches; basil for fatigue; neroli and lavender for insomnia; lemongrass for premenstrual syndrome; and clary sage and rose for depression.

Guidelines for taking herbs
If you're interested in herbal remedies, consult a trained herbalist, but also bear the following points in mind:

- Always use herbs in moderation.
- Stop using them if you experience any side-effects.
- Assess each herb's efficacy over a week or so.
- Start by taking an herb in tea form. Increase the amount from half a cup a day to several cups over a period of a week.
- If you're taking medication, check with your doctor before taking an herbal remedy.
- Don't defer seeking medical advice because you are using an herbal remedy.

WHAT CAN I DO?

A good diet is as important in maintaining health during and after menopause as at any other time of your life. In particular, calcium levels and vitamin D need to be kept up after menopause to avoid thinning and brittle bones – a condition that can lead to osteoporosis.

Never view yourself as over the hill. Keep up your self-respect and self-assurance with your work, or retrain or get involved in voluntary activities. This is often the time in your life when your children leave home, adding extra stress when you may be least capable of coping with it.

On the other hand, many women experience a new lease on life once they are freed of reproductive responsibilities. We hear all the time about women who really come into their own in middle age. Those women who have a positive view of menopause suffer fewer symptoms less seriously. Remember that it marks the end of one phase of your life and the beginning of another. It should not be a time for sadness and regret; in fact, it should be a time for looking forward to enjoying new interests and new experiences.

SEE ALSO:
Cervical Smear, *page 71*
Ectopic Pregnancy, *page 68*
Hysterectomy, *page 79*
Ovarian Cancer, *page 44*

GENITAL PROBLEMS

Just because a woman's genitalia are less exposed
than a man's does not mean that they are
necessarily better protected. Problems can and
do occur – from minor ailments, such as pruritis
vulvae or thrush, to much more serious diseases,
such as cervical cancer. These conditions and the other
common problems that can affect this area of the
body are described in detail in the pages that follow,
with the emphasis on self-help wherever possible.
Practical advice is also given about seeking medical
assistance, when this recourse is more appropriate.

PRURITIS VULVAE

Pruritis vulvae is the name given to an intense itching around the genital organs and rectum, when no obvious cause can be found. The itching often leads to scratching to relieve the irritation, and the cycle becomes difficult to break. If you end up scratching repeatedly for several days, the condition may become chronic, causing a thickening of the vulval skin.

There are no dangers directly associated with pruritis vulvae itself, but if white patches of abnormal skin (leukoplakia), develop in the irritated area, there is a slightly increased risk of developing cancer of the vulva.

SYMPTOMS

- *Intense itchiness of the vulva*
- *Urgent need to scratch*
- *Sensitive skin in the vulval area*
- *Dryness and scaling*
- *Scalding and burning when urinating – scratching causes minute tears, and urine irritates these abrasions*

WHAT CAUSES IT?

The most common cause of pruritis vulvae is an increasing or decreasing supply of the female hormones, estrogen and progesterone. For this reason, pregnant women and young girls approaching puberty, both of whom have increasing levels, are susceptible, while in older women, it is a direct consequence of menopause, when the supply of hormones decreases.

Other possible causes include diabetes, and an allergy to talcum powder, vaginal deodorants, or to nylon panty hose.

If none of these factors apply, the reason for the itching could be emotional – anxiety about a sexual involvement, perhaps, or even a lack of confidence in relationships.

When the itching is accompanied by a thick discharge, the cause could be a vaginal infection such as **thrush**.

SHOULD I SEE THE DOCTOR?

If the itching persists and you are unable to resist scratching, see your doctor as soon as possible. If you try the self-help measures suggested below, and there is no improvement in a week or so, see your doctor.

WHAT MIGHT THE DOCTOR DO?

- For any skin symptoms, your doctor may suggest a course of antihistamine pills to reduce the itching sensation, and a mild sleeping pill, particularly if the itchiness is more severe during the night and causes bouts of insomnia.
- Your doctor may recommend a steroid or hormone cream to be applied to the affected area to relieve irritation.
- If you are over 45, your doctor may suggest that you have some form of HRT, such as estrogen pessaries or creams, to alleviate the problem.

WHAT CAN I DO?

- If the genital area is dry, use an emollient cream to keep the skin well lubricated.
- Cut down on the amount of soap used when washing the area, and avoid hot baths; these overheat the skin, which sets off the itchiness. Have a shower instead.
- Avoid possible irritants, such as scented soaps, douches, talcum powder, vaginal deodorants, and bath oils, and wear cotton or natural-fiber briefs. Wash with warm water after urinating.
- Use a lubricant, such as a water-soluble jelly, during sex.
- Never put antiseptics in the bath water.

SEE ALSO:
Menopause, *page 18*
Painful Intercourse, *page 48*
Thrush, *page 24*
Vaginal Discharge, *page 23*

VAGINAL DISCHARGE

The vagina is kept clean and moist by secretions (discharge) from its lining, and in menstruating women they change their character during each monthly cycle due to the influence of fluctuating hormones. In the first half of the cycle, under the influence of estrogen, the vaginal discharge is clear, thin, and stretchy. After ovulation, it becomes thick, opaque, and rubbery. This change denotes ovulation.

The hormonal changes that occur during pregnancy also affect your discharge and it becomes thick and white.

The amount of vaginal secretions increases with sexual excitement to lubricate the vagina in preparation for sexual intercourse.

Abnormal vaginal discharge is different in color, consistency, and smell from normal discharge and there may be other symptoms, such as soreness and itching. In general terms, any symptoms that accompany abnormal vaginal discharge, such as burning, a rash, and bleeding, should be investigated as soon as possible.

If you cannot make a diagnosis from the information given below, see your doctor.

NATURE OF THE DISCHARGE	PROBABLE CAUSE
There is an increase in your normal secretions	You may be pregnant, have just started taking oral contraceptives, or have recently had an IUD fitted. This is normal and nothing to worry about (see **Contraception**, p. 14).
It is thick and white and your vulva is itchy	This could be **thrush** (see p. 24), a fungal infection of the vagina. Thrush is more common during pregnancy or if you are taking an antibiotic medication for any reason.
The discharge is greenish yellow and has an unpleasant smell	This could be **trichomoniasis** (see p. 25), or perhaps you have forgotten to remove a tampon or your diaphragm.
You notice a slight discharge, and your sexual partner has sores on his genitals	This could be a cervical infection, possibly due to a sexually transmitted disease such as **gonorrhea** (see p. 55).
The discharge is brown, like blood, and usually follows intercourse	This is probably cervical erosion; see your doctor.
The discharge is spotted with blood, either midperiod or following intercourse	This could be a polyp on the cervix; see your doctor.

THRUSH

This is a common infection caused by a fungus, *Candida albicans*, that lives in the digestive tract and is usually kept under control by other bacteria.

If thrush appears in the mouth it is known as oral thrush. If you attempt to wipe away the creamy-yellow or white patches in the mouth, red sore patches are left.

The presence of *Candida albicans* in the vagina often causes a thick "cottage cheese" discharge and itchiness. It is referred to as a vaginal yeast infection.

SYMPTOMS

- *For vaginal thrush, a thick white curdy discharge with soreness and irritation of the vulva*
- *Red rash around the anus which can extend down to the thighs*
- *Urine may burn or irritate the area*
- *Pain during sexual intercourse*
- *For oral thrush, creamy-yellow or white patches inside the mouth that adhere to the mucous membrane*

WHAT CAUSES IT?

For thrush to infect a woman, the conditions in her vagina need to be unbalanced, as the vagina is usually too acid for thrush to thrive. But in some circumstances the acid levels may be lowered; for example, vaginal deodorants can destroy the natural bacteria that prevent the overgrowth of the fungus. A course of antibiotics also alters the natural balance; resistance is low after illness anyway. Diabetics are often affected, as are women with altered hormonal levels (during pregnancy and premenstrually) and women who are using oral contraceptives.

SHOULD I SEE THE DOCTOR?

See your doctor immediately after you notice any of the symptoms of thrush, and refrain from sexual intercourse until you have been treated.

WHAT MIGHT THE DOCTOR DO?

- Your doctor may take a swab of discharge to check that the initial diagnosis is accurate and what treatment is appropriate.
- In most cases of vaginal thrush, she will prescribe antifungal pessaries and soothing ointment, such as clotrimazole, immediately to give you relief from the symptoms. Treatment can take from a day to two weeks. She will also recommend similar treatment for your partner or partners, to prevent reinfection.

WHAT CAN I DO?

- Take the complete course of treatment and return to your doctor if the infection recurs.
- Try not to scratch because the fungus can be spread by hand. Constant scratching will also cause toughening of the skin.
- Some women gain short-term relief by applying plain yogurt to the genital area. Leave it for at least two hours – you can insert it on a tampon to prevent it from leaking out.
- Don't apply anything containing a local anesthetic. It may bring instant relief but it may cause a local allergy too.
- The thrush fungus likes warm, moist conditions, so folds of fat around your groin may be a reason for recurrent vaginal thrush. You may be able to reduce this recurrence by losing weight.
- Always wipe your anus from the front to the back to prevent infection from stools from entering your vagina.
- Wear natural fibers – cotton or silk – next to your genital area if possible. Avoid nylon panty hose and briefs because they don't "breathe" and they give the fungus warm conditions for growth.

SEE ALSO:
Painful Intercourse, *page 48*
Pruritis Vulvae, *page 22*
Trichomoniasis, *page 25*
Vaginal Discharge, *page 23*

TRICHOMONIASIS

Trichomoniasis is an infection caused by a very small one-celled organism (*Trichomonas vaginalis*), which affects the vagina, cervix, urethra, and bladder. The symptoms are similar to those of **thrush**, except that the discharge is green and has an offensive smell. It is contagious, and is usually transmitted sexually, although it can occasionally be caught indirectly from items such as damp towels. The most common time of infection is just after a menstrual period.

SYMPTOMS

- *Offensive-smelling, yellowish-green, bubbly vaginal discharge*
- *Itching of the vagina and perineum (the area between the legs behind the genitals and in front of the anus)*
- *Burning sensation when urinating*
- *Symptoms of cystitis if the bladder is affected*

SHOULD I SEE THE DOCTOR?

If you suspect that you may be infected, see your doctor as soon as possible for an accurate diagnosis, and refrain from sexual intercourse until the doctor tells you it is safe. Let your partner know as soon as possible that you may have a sexually transmitted infection and that treatment might be necessary for him too.

WHAT MIGHT THE DOCTOR DO?

- Your doctor will probably take a sample of the discharge for laboratory analysis. This is important because some other sexually transmitted disease may be diagnosed too, and also because the drugs used to cure trichomoniasis are strong and should not be overprescribed. Give your doctor full details of your medical history.
- Normal treatment is by antibacterial drugs of the metronidazole family, such as Flagyl. These drugs can sometimes produce side-effects, such as nausea and abdominal pain, and they should not be taken by pregnant or breast-feeding women. A normal course of antibacterial medication will last between five and ten days.

WHAT CAN I DO?

- Take the full course of pills as prescribed and do not drink alcohol while you are taking them. If a second course is necessary, you should have a blood count first to check that your blood is normal.
- As with other vaginal infections, practice good hygiene and avoid vaginal deodorants, douches, and tampons.
- Wear natural fibers, such as cotton or silk, next to your skin.
- Don't have sexual intercourse until you have been cured of the infection.
- Provide the names and addresses of your sexual partners so that they can be identified and have treatment too.

SEE ALSO:

Cystitis, *page 28*
Sexually Transmitted Diseases, *page 51*
Thrush, *page 24*

CERVICAL CANCER

Cancer of the cervix is the third most common female cancer in the US (lung cancer is the most common cancer in women, followed by breast cancer). This cancer is becoming more common, particularly among young women.

Cervical cancer is the ninth most deadly form of cancer in the US, and each year approximately one-quarter of the women with cervical cancer die. However, precancerous changes in the cervix can be detected by regular **cervical smear** (Pap smear) tests and, if caught at this early stage, are often treated successfully. Since cervical cancer does not have any symptoms in its early stages, it is detected only by routine screening. As the importance of annual Pap smears has become understood, the death rate has declined.

Cervical cancer has a preinvasive stage during which time it may grow but not spread. Since this preinvasive stage may last for several years, any woman who has regular smear tests should be identified early enough for the cancer to be totally removed by simply taking out the tissue from the cervix.

SYMPTOMS

- *In its early precancerous stages (CIN I and II – see p. 27), there are no symptoms*
- *By CIN III or Stage 1, ulceration of the cervix is visible when the vagina is examined*
- *By stage 1 or 2, intermenstrual bleeding, spotting after intercourse or after menopause*
- *Offensive vaginal discharge*

WHAT CAUSES IT?

It is thought that sexual activity plays a part in causing cancer of the cervix because the lining cells of the cervix are vulnerable in adolescence. Frequent intercourse during this time, especially with several different partners, may initiate the cancer process.

The inference is that there is a carcinogenic component in seminal fluid. This may account for the higher incidence of cancer among young women, since sexual intercourse is occurring earlier in women's lives. This is backed up by looking at certain religious groups such as Orthodox Jewish and Moslem women. Cervical cancer is much rarer among these women, probably because the men are circumcised and extramarital intercourse is less common. Women whose mothers took DES (a drug to prevent recurrent miscarriages) in pregnancy are among others with a particularly high risk.

WHAT IS THE MEDICAL TREATMENT?

- All stages of CIN (cervical intrapithelial neoplasia) should be treated, although some doctors adopt a "wait and see" approach, involving repeat smear tests for early CIN and changes that might be caused by infection with **genital warts**.
- Treatment of CIN involves performing a **colposcopy** usually in the outpatient department, when the cervix is viewed with a special microscope. Areas with abnormal cells may be identified and, if necessary, a biopsy may be taken to examine the tissue.
- Following a colposcopy a woman will either be reassured and a follow-up smear arranged, or treated further.

WHAT IS THE SURGICAL TREATMENT?

- Surgical treatment of CIN involves removing the precancerous tissue under a local anesthetic with a laser, or freezing, or burning away the tissue with an electric current (LLETZ – large loop excision of the transformation zone).
- Occasionally, a general anesthetic is required for a **cone biopsy**. This may be done with a scalpel or a laser beam. After the tissue is examined microscopically, doctors decide if you require any further treatment.

• The treatment of full-blown cancer of the cervix depends on the stage that the disease is at. Treatment may involve either surgery or radiation therapy, or both. As a general rule, however, radiation therapy is more often used for older women and surgery for younger, fitter patients, irrespective of the stage of the disease.

• Surgery involves removing affected tissue. A radical (Wertheim's) **hysterectomy** is most often performed. This involves removing the uterus and the surrounding tissue, including some lymph nodes.

• If retaining your fertility is important, trachylectomy, or removal of the cervix, may be performed, although this is rare.

• If there is a recurrence of the cancer following radiation therapy, major surgery involving removal of the bladder or bowel may be necessary.

HOW IS RADIATION THERAPY USED?

Nearly half the cases of cervical cancer are treated with radiation therapy. The aim is to give a fatal dose of radiation to the center

STAGES OF CERVICAL PRECANCER AND CANCER

For precancer
• The mildest stage, known as mild dysplasia or CIN I
• More severe inflammation called moderate dysplasia or CIN II
• Severe dysplasia, with or without non-invasive carcinoma in situ, or CIN III

For cancer
• Stage 1: Cancer confined to the cervix
• Stage 2: Cancer extends beyond the cervix to involve the upper third of the vagina and/or lateral tissue immediately surrounding the cervix
• Stage 3: Cancer extends to the lower third of the vagina and/or pelvic side wall
• Stage 4: Cancer extends beyond the pelvis and/or involves the bladder or rectum

of the cancer. Radiation also kills those parts of the growth that were invading other areas. In studies comparing women who had radiation therapy with those who had radical surgery, the survival rate after five years was about the same, so it's well worth discussing the options fully with your doctor.

WHAT CAN I DO?

• You will be required to have regular checks over the next five years or so to make sure the cancer has not spread.

• You will almost certainly not be able to have any more children and, if you had your ovaries removed, you will go through a premature menopause. If this causes you to suffer unpleasant symptoms, see your doctor for treatment.

• If you maintain regular appointments for smear tests, any cancer will be caught at a time when chances of a cure are high. Even if cancerous cells are found, you should take an interest in the disease and cooperate with your medical advisers as much as possible to fight it. Cancer cures do depend to a certain extent on the determination of the patient to conquer the disease.

SEE ALSO:
Cervical Smear, *page 71*
Colposcopy, *page 72*
Cone Biopsy, *page 81*
Genital Warts, *page 53*
Hysterectomy, *page 79*
Sexually Transmitted Diseases, *page 51*

CYSTITIS

Cystitis is an inflammation of the bladder, which may be the result of an infection or bruising after athletic sex.

The most common symptom is a frequent urge to urinate, with only a small flow occurring each time; this is nearly always accompanied by severe pain, which worsens when urination is completed. Other symptoms that may occur include smelly or blood-stained urine, fever, occasional chills, and lower abdominal pain.

Many of the symptoms of cystitis can apply to unrelated problems and other vaginal diseases. For instance, a strong yellow- to orange-colored urine, even one with a strong smell, is not necessarily indicative of cystitis, or indeed any other infection. It is just as likely to be a symptom of dehydration, either due to vomiting or sweating profusely, or simply because you have not drunk enough fluid. Occasionally, food such as asparagus, if eaten in large quantities, can also cause urine to change color.

Cystitis is very common, annoying, and inconvenient, but it does not endanger general health. Most women have it at some time in their lives. It is particularly common during pregnancy: in the first few months, when the urethra relaxes under the influence of the hormone progesterone, and infections spread more easily, and later on when the pressure of the enlarging uterus may cause a small amount of urine to remain in the bladder after urination. This becomes stagnant and the lack of flow may encourage bacteria to multiply, which results in cystitis.

WHAT CAUSES IT?

The most common infecting organism is *E. coli,* a bacterium that normally lives in the bowel and around the anus and only causes problems when it spreads up the urethra into the bladder. Women are more prone to cystitis than men because their urethra is shorter than that of men.

The type of cystitis known as "honeymoon cystitis" is caused by unusual amounts of frequent, strenuous sexual intercourse, which can bruise the urethra.

Occasionally, infection can be caused by other things, such as the use of antiseptics in bathwater, or the overzealous use of vaginal deodorants or douches.

As women become older and reach menopause, a shortage of estrogen and progesterone can lead to the thinning of all genital organs and the perineum (the area between the genitals and the anus), and in some unexplained way this can contribute to a menopausal type of cystitis. **Prolapse** of the front of the vaginal wall may also be a cause because of poor urinary flow and stagnating urine.

If a woman needs an indwelling catheter, as she might after an operation or if she suffers from incontinence due to a disease such as multiple sclerosis, for example, then an infection could occur. This rarely happens, however, as long as the catheter is inserted and removed correctly using a sterile technique.

SYMPTOMS

- *The urgent need to urinate frequently though only a small amount may be passed each time*
- *A severe dragging-down pain, usually in the front of the abdomen but quite often radiating up the flanks and to the back*
- *A burning or stinging sensation while urinating*
- *A severe pain on urinating*
- *The passage of blood in the urine which may be pink, red, or simply streaked with blood*
- *The urge to get up several times in the night to empty your bladder even though there may be very little urine present*

Contrary to popular belief, dirty toilet habits do not *per se* cause cystitis, although you should always wipe yourself from the front to the back.

SHOULD I SEE THE DOCTOR?

If the self-help measures listed below don't bring relief, seek help from your doctor as soon as possible.

WHAT MIGHT THE DOCTOR DO?

• Your doctor may take a urine specimen to confirm which bacterium is causing your symptoms so that she can gauge its sensitivity to a range of antibiotic drugs, the normal treatment for cystitis.

• As soon as the specimen has been analyzed, she can start you on a course of antibiotics, usually a penicillin derivative. It's absolutely essential that you take the full course of treatment even if your symptoms subside completely within 24 hours (they often do; some sufferers report complete relief after about only two hours). If you do not do so, the infecting organisms may become resistant to antibiotics and your cystitis can become chronic. If this happens, it can be exceedingly difficult to eradicate.

• If your cystitis does not respond to treatment, your doctor may recommend a full hospital investigation to see whether or not there is any predisposing internal cause.

• If investigation shows no trace of a bacterium, you may be suffering from an irritable bladder, which is often caused by emotional factors.

WHAT CAN I DO?

• Drink plenty of fluids at the first sign of the symptoms. It's important to get urine flowing fast to flush out the bladder, so try to drink the equivalent of a glass of water every half hour.

• Make your urine alkaline by adding a little baking soda to your drinks. You will find that alkalinizing your urine eases bladder pain quite considerably.

• For pain relief, take acetaminophen every four hours. A warm pad or wrapped-up hot water bottle on the front of the abdomen may also help.

• Drink cranberry juice, which is a urinary antiseptic.

TO PREVENT A RECURRENCE

• Drink plenty of water at all times.

• At the first symptom, increase your water intake and alkalinize your urine by adding a little baking soda to your drinks. (Don't continue this for too long; you could have unpleasant side effects, such as gas.)

• If you are having sex frequently, drink a lot of fluid to keep the urine flowing. Urinate before and after sexual intercourse.

• Use tampons instead of sanitary napkins since they are less likely to allow bacteria to thrive; some women find, however, that tampons irritate the bladder further.

• If you suspect that wearing a diaphragm is a contributory cause, ask about another form of contraception.

• Wear cotton briefs or cotton liners.

• Don't use antiseptics in the bathwater, and don't use vaginal douches or deodorants.

• Don't be obsessive about washing your perineum with soap and water. Using a bidet, if you have one, after moving your bowels is a good idea so that you avoid contamination of the vagina and urethra from the rectum.

• Depending on the medicines prescribed by your doctor, you can make them more effective by adjusting the acidity or alkalinity of your urine. Ask your doctor what your antibiotic is. For example, tetracycline is more effective if your urine is acidic, so drink plenty of cranberry juice while you are taking it.

SEE ALSO:

Contraception, *page 14*
Incontinence, *page 32*
Menopause, *page 18*
Prolapse, *page 30*

PROLAPSE

Another name for prolapse is "pelvic relaxation." Vaginal wall prolapse occurs when the pelvic muscles become weakened and allow one or several pelvic organs to drop down the vagina. Pelvic organs, including the bladder, rectum, and urethra, can prolapse into the vagina, but the most commonly affected organ is the uterus. The vaginal wall is pushed down by the unsupported and descending uterus and, depending on the severity, the cervix may protrude from the vulva.

If the rectum bulges into the back of the vaginal wall, it is called a *rectocele*; when the urethra bulges into the front of the vaginal wall, it is known as a *urethrocele*; while if the bladder drops into the front of the vaginal wall, it is called a *cystocele*.

Prolapse tends to occur in older women, and is much more common in those who have had children.

WHAT CAUSES IT?

Pelvic floor muscles can weaken with age, but prolapse is nearly always caused by earlier injury to the pelvic floor muscles, cervix, or supporting tissue of the uterus during labor, especially if you had a rapid delivery, were allowed to go on too long in labor, or if your babies were large.

SYMPTOMS
- *Severe backache*
- *Intense pain during sexual intercourse or inability to achieve orgasm if the vagina is slack*
- *Stress incontinence*
- *For uterine prolapse, a dragging down feeling in the pelvis*
- *For urethrocele, frequency of urination*
- *For cystocele, frequency of urination and cystitis-type symptoms of pain and burning when urinating*
- *For rectocele, discomfort on moving the bowels, difficulty in defecating*

SHOULD I SEE THE DOCTOR?

If your prolapse is accompanied by severe backache or pelvic discomfort, you should consult your doctor as soon as possible.

WHAT MIGHT THE DOCTOR DO?

- Your doctor will give you an internal pelvic examination to confirm a prolapse and to determine which type you have.
- She will ask you about your deliveries – for example if your babies were larger than normal, and if the second stage of labor lasted a long time.
- Being overweight can cause the prolapse to be more troublesome, so your doctor will advise you to lose excess weight.
- If you have a severe prolapse, your doctor may recommend surgery. This is rarely absolutely necessary, but will improve your quality of life by maintaining urinary continence and improving sexual enjoyment.
- For mild prolapse a doctor will recommend Kegel exercises (see opposite). For older women who are too frail for surgery, there are vaginal rings to help support the vaginal walls or uterus. You may be fitted with a ring or sponge pessary that is placed high in the vagina; these, however, can erode internal tissues so should not be worn for long periods.

SURGICAL TREATMENT

- Surgery is carried out to improve quality of life. If there are any reasons why surgery may not be a good idea, for example due to extreme frailty, it is best avoided and nonsurgical methods employed to control the symptoms. Very rarely, an anterior repair may result in urinary incontinence, and a posterior repair may sometimes result in uncomfortable or painful intercourse.
- Most prolapse repairs are performed through the vagina and involve a general anesthetic. Occasionally the operation may be performed under an epidural anesthetic, especially if the patient is old and infirm.

PELVIC FLOOR MUSCLES

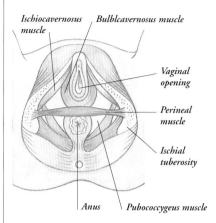

Ischiocavernosus muscle

Bulblcavernosus muscle

Vaginal opening

Perineal muscle

Ischial tuberosity

Anus

Pubococcygeus muscle

Pelvic floor muscles
Supporting the bowel, bladder, and uterus, these muscles can become stretched during pregnancy owing to the weight of the fetus.

KEGEL EXERCISES

You should do this routine at least five or six times a day. If you find it difficult to set aside time specifically for it, then do it when urinating. If you are pregnant, you should only do these exercises as a test occasionally; it is not advisable to do them all the time.
• First, identify the muscles you are going to use. The easiest way to do this is to stop the flow of urine in midstream when you empty your bladder.
• Now, draw up these muscles in the same way or as if you were holding a tampon in place, hold for a count of five, and relax.
• Repeat this process at least five times or as often as you can – more if you have just had a baby.
• After a while, you could repeat the process as above, but hold for a longer count before relaxing.

• The repair involves making an incision in the wall of the vagina and strengthening the tissues that have become weakened using buttressing sutures (stitches). Any excess or stretched tissue is removed from the vaginal walls and the incision is closed using stitches that are absorbed by the body.
• Following the operation, the vagina is packed with gauze, which remains in place for one or two days. A catheter is inserted into the bladder during the operation to help drain urine. It is common to have some discharge from the vagina for a few days following surgery.
• You will probably stay in the hospital for five to seven days. An outpatient appointment is usually made six weeks later, after which sexual intercourse can be resumed if there are no problems.
• For difficult-to-treat or recurrent prolapse, an abdominal operation is occasionally carried out to strengthen the walls of the vagina.

WHAT CAN I DO?

• If you suffer from backache, try to avoid standing for long periods at a time. Wear a tight girdle to counteract any dragging feeling you may have in your pelvis.
• If you are having difficulty with sexual intercourse, you and your partner may need to explore alternative ways of achieving sexual pleasure.
• Wear panty liners if you are bothered by leakage of urine (stress incontinence). If it becomes worse, see your doctor.
• The most important preventative treatment is being conscientious about doing pelvic floor exercises regularly during pregnancy and especially after the birth of your baby, whether you have stitches or not.

SEE ALSO:
Cystitis, *page 28*
Hysterectomy, *page 79*
Incontinence, *page 32*
Painful Intercourse, *page 48*

INCONTINENCE

Incontinence is the involuntary leakage of urine when you are unable to control your bladder. Many women suffer from occasional bouts of incontinence from their middle twenties onward, particularly if they have borne children, and most older women suffer from it from time to time to a greater or lesser degree.

SYMPTOMS
- *Inability to control your bladder, particularly when you exert pressure on the abdominal muscles*
- *Frequency of urination, even when your bladder is not full*
- *Urgency, even when your bladder is not full*

WHAT CAUSES IT?

There are three major causes of incontinence in women. In the aftermath of pregnancy, the pelvic and perineal tissues can become so stretched that a **prolapse** of the vaginal wall occurs. If even a very small part of the urethra or bladder accompanies the prolapse, this nearly always leads to urinary symptoms of some kind or other, whether it is urgency, hesitancy, frequency, and/or pain.

As a woman becomes older, the exit valve from the bladder can weaken slightly. (This is not uncommon during pregnancy, in fact, but goes away after delivery.)

Urine may also leak away when pressure inside the abdominal cavity is increased when, for example, we sneeze, cough, strain to open our bowels, or lift a heavy weight. This is called stress incontinence.

If the muscles of the bladder wall become oversensitive to the presence of urine in the bladder, they respond by contracting uncontrollably and trying to empty the bladder even when there are only small quantities of urine present. This is sometimes called irritable bladder.

SHOULD I SEE THE DOCTOR?

You should seek help as soon as the symptoms of incontinence appear. The earlier it is treated, the less likely it is that weaknesses will persist and the condition become chronic. Both stress incontinence and irritable bladder can be treated successfully.

WHAT MIGHT THE DOCTOR DO?

- Your doctor will take a midstream urine sample to check whether there is any urinary tract infection, such as **cystitis**, present. She may also refer you for a special X ray of your bladder.
- She will advise you to strengthen your pelvic floor muscles by doing Kegel exercises (see p. 31). Since obesity weakens the pelvic floor, if you are overweight you may be advised to consult a dietitian, or to exercise in order to reduce your weight.
- Recommended treatment for prolapse involves wearing a special ring or sponge in your vagina during the day.
- If treatment for stress incontinence fails to work, your doctor will advise you to have a surgical operation to tighten up your pelvic floor muscles.
- If you are suffering from an irritable bladder, she may encourage you to hold on to urine for as long as possible to strengthen the bladder muscles, or she may suggest a drug to relax them. If neither of these work, she may advise a surgical operation to stretch the urethra.

WHAT CAN I DO?

Practice Kegel exercises regularly (see p. 31) to regain muscle control, and therefore, bladder control.

SEE ALSO:
Cystitis, *page 28*
Prolapse, *page 30*

MENSTRUAL PROBLEMS

Menstruation is a normal part of a woman's life. Most women menstruate for well over 30 years, from their early teens to their late 40s or early 50s. Most of the time, menstrual periods occur in a regular pattern and are trouble-free, but many women experience complaints at some point. The most common disorders are painful periods (dysmenorrhea) and premenstrual syndrome. Less common but potentially more serious conditions include vaginal bleeding between periods and amenorrhea (no periods); all these and more are described here, with the emphasis on what can be done to cure or alleviate them.

PREMENSTRUAL SYNDROME

More widely known as PMS, this disorder affects about 75 percent of all women emotionally, mentally, and physically in the days prior to menstruation. The most common symptoms are irritability, depression, fatigue, and fluid retention.

SYMPTOMS

- *Fluid retention – with heavy breasts, thickened waistline, puffy face, hands, and feet, causing headaches and pain especially in the breasts and abdomen*
- *Changes in mood – irritability, bad temper, tearfulness*
- *Depression, often leading to suicidal feelings and violence toward oneself and others*

WHAT CAUSES IT?

The exact cause is still not known but it is likely that the symptoms are in some way linked with falling levels of the female hormones, estrogen and progesterone, in the days just prior to menstruation.

SHOULD I SEE THE DOCTOR?

If your symptoms are severe enough to disturb your normal life every month and self-help measures don't alleviate them, contact your doctor as soon as possible.

WHAT MIGHT THE DOCTOR DO?

- Your doctor will question you about the symptoms and possibly ask you to record them over several months.
- He may suggest progesterone therapy, probably in pessary or suppository form, on a trial basis. This can help some women, although there is no convincing evidence to suggest that all women would benefit from it. Treatment should start four days before you expect symptoms.
- If you suffer from fluid retention, he may offer you a diuretic medication. These are taken for about ten days before your period.

- Your doctor may offer antidepressant medicines or suggest that you take the oral contraceptive pill, both of which are known to relieve symptoms in some women.

WHAT CAN I DO?

- Keep a diary of when your symptoms occur so that you can start the treatment that works for you at the appropriate time.
- Eat little and often to keep your strength up and, if you are constipated, eat plenty of high-fiber foods.
- If you are prescribed a diuretic, you will urinate much more often and possibly flush important minerals out of your system, so watch your diet by increasing your intake of foods rich in minerals such as potassium (fruits, seafoods, nuts, and beans) and by taking extra amounts of Vitamins C and B, either in your diet or as supplements.
- To help prevent fluid retention, cut salt out of your diet as much as you can. Salt absorbs water and therefore increases the possibility of retention.
- Get plenty of rest to prevent exhaustion, and try to limit stressful situations if this is at all possible.
- Talk about your feelings to anyone who will listen, and make sure your close family knows to what extent you are affected.
- For pain such as that associated with **dysmenorrhea**, try aspirin, which will inhibit prostaglandin production. Excessive prostaglandin is believed to be the cause of the contraction-like pains experienced during menstruation.
- Exercise such as swimming and walking, deep breathing, and relaxation techniques can all be helpful in bringing relief from tension and insomnia.

SEE ALSO:
Dysmenorrhea, *page 37*

AMENORRHEA

Amenorrhea is the medical term for an absence of menstrual periods. It is described as *primary* if they have never started, and *secondary*, when normal menstruation is interrupted for four months or more. Amenorrhea does not necessarily mean you are ill; it does usually mean that you are not producing eggs and so cannot conceive.

SYMPTOMS

- *For primary amenorrhea, a failure to start menstruation and pubertal development – no development of sexual characteristics such as body hair, breasts, and pelvic broadening*
- *For secondary amenorrhea, periods stop suddenly or gradually cease with each successive month until the flow dries up*

WHAT CAUSES IT?

Primary amenorrhea is usually due to late onset of puberty, although it can also be caused by a disorder of the reproductive or hormonal system. The most common reason for secondary amenorrhea is pregnancy. If the hormonal balance is interrupted for any other reason, however, menstrual periods may stop. So, for example, many women who breast-feed find that their periods do not start again until they wean their babies.

More seriously, amenorrhea can be a side-effect of being grossly underweight, such as with anorexia nervosa. This will be suspected if your weight is as much as 26lb (12kg) below average for your height and frame. Stress, chronic ailments such as thyroid disease, and long-term medication with drugs such as tranquilizers and anti-depressants can also cause amenorrhea, as can excessive physical training.

Amenorrhea is, of course, a permanent condition after menopause, or if you undergo a **hysterectomy** with removal of your ovaries.

SHOULD I SEE THE DOCTOR?

The tendency to start menstruation late may be inherited, so if your mother started her periods late, don't worry if you aren't developing at the same rate as your friends. However, if you are 16 and have not yet menstruated, contact your doctor to check that there is no abnormality. If your periods suddenly stop, pregnancy could be the cause, so do a pregnancy test first before contacting him. See your doctor if your periods have been absent for six months and you are not pregnant or menopausal.

WHAT MIGHT THE DOCTOR DO?

- If you have never had a menstrual period, your doctor will probably give you a physical examination and take a blood sample to measure the level of pituitary hormones. (The pituitary hormones include those responsible for menstruation.)
- With secondary amenorrhea, once pregnancy is excluded, you should receive a full medical examination by a specialist, and if you are taking any long-term medications, these should be checked out and stopped if necessary.
- Your doctor may arrange for you to have an X ray to make sure that your pituitary gland is healthy.
- If you are not ovulating, and not pregnant, he may suggest that you take a course of fertility drugs or pituitary hormones.

WHAT CAN I DO?

- The lack of periods is not dangerous and in most cases there is no cause for alarm; be patient and they will start up naturally.
- You may need to change your lifestyle to correct any dietary or physical problems, if these are the cause.

SEE ALSO:
Hysterectomy, *page 79*
Menopause, *page 18*

ABNORMAL BLEEDING

All women bleed from the vagina during menstruation. Any change in your normal cycle, however, or bleeding between periods should be treated with suspicion.

If you notice any bloody discharge during pregnancy, call your doctor, lie down, and wait. The cause will depend on whether you are in early or late pregnancy.

If you are postmenopausal, and you know that your periods have definitely stopped, remember that vaginal bleeding is not normal unless you are taking combined estrogen-progestogen HRT.

If you are unable to make a diagnosis from the information listed here, consult your doctor.

NATURE OF THE BLEEDING	PROBABLE CAUSE
Irregular bleeding, particularly if you are younger than 15 or older than 45	Irregular bleeding can be the result of hormonal changes. An occasional irregularity may not be cause for concern, but see your doctor if the cycle hasn't settled down after two months.
Your periods become unusually heavy	This is known as **menorrhagia** (see p. 38). You may suffer from anemia if you lose a lot of blood every month. See your doctor.
Bleeding following intercourse	This could be cervical erosion. Go to your doctor for a **cervical smear** test (see p. 71).
Bleeding during pregnancy	This might be a **miscarriage** (see p. 66), or if there is severe abdominal pain, an **ectopic pregnancy** (see p. 68). Call the doctor immediately.
Bleeding is only spotting, and you're on oral contraceptives	This may be breakthrough bleeding. If it is bothersome, see your doctor; you may want to change your method of contraception.
Breakthrough bleeding after you have had an IUD fitted	See your doctor or go to the family planning clinic.
Excessive bleeding during the menopausal years	During menopause, your menstrual periods may change in character, but if they are heavy, see your doctor at once.

DYSMENORRHEA

Dysmenorrhea is the medical name for menstrual periods accompanied by cramps and pain. There are two different types: *primary*, which is painful periods experienced within three years of the onset of menstruation and in which there is no underlying disease to account for it; and *secondary*, which is a symptom of an underlying gynecological disease such as **endometriosis** or **fibroids**.

SYMPTOMS
- *Violent abdominal cramps lasting up to three days*
- *Diarrhea*
- *Frequency of urination*
- *Sweating*
- *Pelvic soreness with the pain radiating down into the upper thighs and into the back*
- *Abdominal distension*
- *Backache*
- *Nausea and vomiting*

WHAT CAUSES IT?

About one third of all menstruating women will experience some pain with their periods. Women who have primary dysmenorrhea produce excessive quantities of the hormone prostaglandin at the time of menstruation and are extremely sensitive to it. Prostaglandin is one of the hormones released during labor and is in part responsible for the uterine contractions. Dysmenorrhea can therefore be seen as a mini-labor with the prostaglandin causing uterine muscle to go into spasm, producing cramplike pain.

SHOULD I SEE THE DOCTOR?

If you have recently begun to menstruate, visit your doctor if pain medication in moderate quantities is not sufficient to dull the pain and you need to spend at least a day in bed each month. If you have been menstruating for three years and the blood flow and pain increase, visit your doctor to confirm that there is no underlying disorder responsible.

WHAT MIGHT THE DOCTOR DO?

- Some doctors may suggest that the pain is psychosomatic, but it isn't. Don't be put off from consulting your doctor by the hope that the pain will pass as you get older or if you have children.
- You should insist on a trial of anti-prostaglandin medicines, which should be taken just prior to, and for the first two to three days of menstruation. The contraceptive pill is often prescribed to relieve dysmenorrhea because it inhibits egg production and alters hormonal balance, so it is a highly effective treatment. The progesterone IUD also helps it.
- If you have developed painful menstrual periods after several years of predictable menstrual characteristics, your doctor will examine you and recommend treatment according to the diagnosis.

WHAT CAN I DO?

- Experiment with herbal teas such as mint or camomile that reduce spasmodic pain.
- Relaxation or special yoga-type exercises can also help to relieve the pain; hot-water bottles, hot baths, and bed rest can all bring relief.
- Nonsteroidal anti-inflammatory medicines and aspirin impede the production of prostaglandins and are, therefore, the best pain medications to take.

SEE ALSO:

Contraception, *page 14*
Endometriosis, *page 40*
Fibroids, *page 41*
Premenstrual Syndrome, *page 34*

MENORRHAGIA

Menorrhagia is the term used to describe menstruation in which blood flow is unusually heavy. It can be a single bout of flooding, a period that goes on for a long time (more than seven days), or very frequent periods so that the blood loss in any given month is excessive. On average only about 2 fl oz (60 ml) of blood is lost during a single period, but sufferers from menorrhagia can lose up to a third more than this.

SYMPTOMS

- *Blood flow during menstruation so rapid and excessive that several sanitary pads must be worn at the same time*
- *Pallor, fatigue, and breathlessness indicating anemia*

WHAT CAUSES IT?

Menorrhagia may be triggered by an imbalance of estrogen and progesterone, which causes the lining of the womb (endometrium) to thicken, with a consequently heavier blood loss as the lining is shed during menstruation. It is common in women approaching **menopause**. The recent fitting of an IUD can cause heavier periods for a few months afterward, and **fibroids** may also cause heavy bleeding because they increase the inner surface of the womb and its lining.

If an excessive rate of flow continues over several days and throughout several menstrual periods, anemia may develop which, if left untreated, could become severe.

SHOULD I SEE THE DOCTOR?

If your periods change and become longer or much heavier than they were, see your doctor to determine the underlying cause.

WHAT MIGHT THE DOCTOR DO?

- Your doctor will examine you for any abnormality of the uterus, such as fibroids, and for signs of anemia.

- He may give you a blood test to determine if you are anemic; if you are, this will be treated with iron supplements.
- If you have an IUD fitted, your doctor may remove it or fit another device if it is not right for you; a progesterone-carrying intrauterine device can be highly effective, for instance.
- If there is no disease of the uterus, he will recommend hormone therapy aimed at preventing buildup of endometrial tissue prior to menstruation. This is often the combined oral contraceptive pill unless you are already on it or it is unsuitable for you, in which case he will prescribe another medication for you.
- If fibroids or some other cause is suspected, you will be given a **hysteroscopy** to scrape out the uterine lining.
- If the menorrhagia is grossly debilitating, your doctor may suggest a **hysterectomy**. You should not agree to have this operation without fully discussing the options with your gynecologist, and then only after careful consideration.

WHAT CAN I DO?

- If you have just one period with heavy bleeding, rest if you can and use extra-absorbant sanitary pads with tampons to minimize embarrassment.
- Increase the iron content in your diet; liver, egg yolks, and dark green leafy vegetables are all rich in iron. To improve the absorption of iron supplements, take them with drinks rich in Vitamin C, such as orange juice. Cooking in iron pots also helps increase the iron content of food.

SEE ALSO:
Contraception, *page 14*
Endometriosis, *page 40*
Fibroids, *page 41*
Hysterectomy, *page 79*
Hysteroscopy, *page 74*
Menopause, *page 18*

PELVIC PROBLEMS

Most of the time our reproductive system functions
smoothly but, particularly during the later years of
menstruation, problems can occur. Some of the conditions
described in the previous chapter, for example, can be
symptoms of pelvic problems such as endometriosis and
fibroids, while a small percentage of women have ovary
problems, from cysts to cancer. All of these can be serious,
but help is available. The most important thing is to
make the most appropriate decisions about your
treatment. The pages that follow give the information
you need to make an informed choice.

ENDOMETRIOSIS

This is a very common condition, defined as the presence of cells from the lining of the uterus at other sites in the pelvis. The principal route of spread is via the fallopian tubes, with implantation of deposits on the ovaries, bowel, bladder, or in the pelvis. The deposits respond to the cyclical changes of the ovarian hormones, so bleeding occurs at the site of implantation when you are menstruating, but the blood cannot escape. The repeated bleeding can cause menstrual pain and painful sexual intercourse as well as generalized pelvic tenderness. Adhesions may form, interfering with ovulation and possibly conception.

SYMPTOMS
- *Heavy or abnormal bleeding*
- *Severe abdominal and pelvic pain, often leading to painful intercourse*
- *Severe cramping pain, starting before the period is due and continuing during menstruation, after which it gradually eases*
- *Occasional urinary or bowel pain, including diarrhea*
- *Fertility problems: difficulty in conceiving a baby*

SHOULD I SEE THE DOCTOR?

If you are in your late twenties and have been unable to conceive, or if you suffer very painful menstrual periods or pain deep in your pelvis during intercourse, you should see your doctor as soon as possible. If you have never suffered from **dysmenorrhea** (painful periods) before, it is very unlikely to develop in your late twenties without a major reason.

WHAT MIGHT THE DOCTOR DO?

- Medical treatment of endometriosis is usually only offered to women who are not trying to conceive; it has not been shown to improve fertility rates.

- The medicines used to treat endometriosis suppress ovulation and menstruation, thus permitting the disease to regress. They include the continuous use of high dose estrogens and/or progestogens or medication to suppress ovarian-stimulating hormones. All these treatments are contraceptive.
- For women wishing to conceive, surgical treatment, usually laparoscopic, includes diathermy (electrical treatment with intense heat) or laser vaporization of the endometriosis deposits, and adhesiolysis (removal of adhesions).
- In vitro fertilization (IVF) should be offered promptly to women trying to conceive who have dense, widespread adhesions that are not amenable to, or recur after, surgery.
- Radical surgery with removal of the uterus and ovaries may be necessary in older patients with advanced disease.

WHAT CAN I DO?

Join a self-help group where you can share your experience with other women and discuss the latest treatments and side-effects of the hormone treatment.

SEE ALSO:
Dysmenorrhea, *page 37*
Fertility Problems, *page 59*
Hysterectomy, *page 79*
Laparoscopy, *page 77*
Menstrual Problems, *page 33*
Painful Intercourse, *page 48*

FIBROIDS

These are benign tumors in the muscle lining the uterine wall. They vary in size and number; they can be anything from the size of a pea to as large as a tennis ball. About one woman in five develops fibroids by the time she is 45 years old.

There is often no reason for concern because the fibroids may never grow large enough to distort the uterus and present symptoms to alarm you. However, if you are having difficulty in conceiving, they may be interfering with your fertility by blocking the fallopian tubes. Large fibroids cause the muscular coating of the uterus to feel lumpy and bumpy to the doctor when he examines your abdomen during routine pelvic examinations.

SYMPTOMS

- *About one quarter of women have no symptoms at all*
- *Very heavy or abnormal menstrual bleeding*
- *Swelling and a feeling of heaviness in the abdomen*
- *Discomfort or pain during intercourse*
- *Pressure on the bladder and bowel, leading to urinary problems and backache*

SHOULD I SEE THE DOCTOR?

If you are having difficulty conceiving, if you have increasing pain or bleeding with your menstrual periods, or if you have any other change in your normal cycle, see your doctor at once.

WHAT MIGHT THE DOCTOR DO?

- Your doctor will first perform a routine pelvic examination and question you about any symptoms you may have experienced.
- If she feels that your condition warrants it, she may then refer you to a gynecologist for further investigation and tests, which will probably include an **ultrasound scan** of your uterus or a **laparoscopy**.

WHAT IS THE TREATMENT?

- Fibroids are treated according to the seriousness of the symptoms and whether you wish to conceive. Once you are past childbearing days, the fibroids usually shrink and disappear anyway.
- If you want children and the fibroids are numerous, your doctor may suggest a **myomectomy**. This removes the fibroids from the uterine lining and leaves the uterus intact and back in its usual shape.
- If the symptoms are difficult and you do not plan to get pregnant in the future, a **hysterectomy** might be advised. This should be considered as a last resort and only after at least two opinions and discussion with your doctors.
- Antiestrogen hormone treatments may be given. These make fibroids shrink, but can only be given for a period of six months because of the risk of osteoporosis, and are only given before a myomectomy.

WHAT CAN I DO?

- Fibroids are the most common reason for hysterectomy operations in the United States, so make sure your condition requires an operation of such a radical nature. If you are suffering from profound anemia, or have unbearable symptoms, obviously you should consider it; otherwise, you should look for alternatives.
- There is a high incidence of **uterine cancer** in women who suffer from benign fibroids, so any unusual bleeding or other irregularity in your menstrual pattern should be investigated immediately.

SEE ALSO:
Hysterectomy, *page 79*
Laparoscopy, *page 77*
Menstruation, *page 10*
Myomectomy, *page 78*
Ultrasound Scan, *page 75*
Uterine Cancer, *page 45*

OVARIAN CYSTS

A cyst is a fluid-filled sac. Ovarian cysts are nearly always benign and a significant proportion of women suffer from them. Benign cysts may be subdivided into two major categories.

Functional cysts are merely large cysts that occur normally during a woman's monthly menstrual cycle. They do not usually cause any problems, although there may be several and they may be present in both ovaries. They rarely grow larger than about 2–3 in (6–8 cm) in diameter and they commonly shrink back to normal size spontaneously.

They are usually detected on routine **ultrasound** screening or **pelvic examination**. Very occasionally a functional cyst may cause the ovary to twist, thereby causing severe abdominal pain. A cyst may also leak, releasing a jellylike material into the abdominal cavity.

The second type of benign ovarian cyst is called a *dermoid cyst*. These are most commonly found in women in their thirties. Dermoid cysts may occasionally be present in both ovaries. They do not usually cause any problems unless they cause the ovary to twist or if the cyst leaks.

Dermoid cysts contain immature cells that are capable of growing into various types of tissue, and it is therefore not uncommon for dermoid cysts to contain bone, teeth, and hair.

Polycystic ovaries create a specific syndrome in women who experience the condition, and this is discussed in detail in the box opposite.

SYMPTOMS

- *Pain during intercourse*
- *Painful, heavy menstrual periods*
- *If a cyst twists or ruptures, it results in severe abdominal pain, nausea, and fever*
- *Urinary problems due to pressure on the bladder*

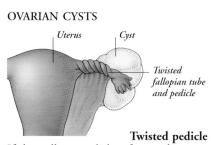

OVARIAN CYSTS

Uterus   *Cyst*

Twisted fallopian tube and pedicle

Twisted pedicle
If the stalk, or pedicle, of a cyst becomes twisted, it cuts off its blood supply and causes sudden, severe abdominal pain.

SHOULD I SEE THE DOCTOR?

While ovarian cysts are small, they produce few symptoms. Many disappear on their own and you may never even know you had them. As they get larger, however, they may cause pain and discomfort and may also affect your menstrual cycle; the severe pain of a twisted ovary requires an emergency operation, so see your doctor as soon as possible if you suffer any of the symptoms detailed in the box on the left.

WHAT MIGHT THE DOCTOR DO?

- Your doctor will examine you both externally and internally in order to assess the size of the ovarian cyst. Further tests will be arranged depending on what your doctor finds, and on your age.
- These tests will probably include an ultrasound examination of your ovaries, plus blood tests and X rays.
- Laparoscopic surgery may be attempted to help diagnose the type of cyst present and, in younger women, to remove the cyst if it is benign.
- In older women, those in whom the cyst is too large to be removed by **laparoscopy**, or where there is a suspicion of malignancy, an abdominal operation will be performed. Both ovaries are always examined and checked during surgery.

POLYCYSTIC OVARIAN SYNDROME

Polycystic ovaries are benign cysts of the ovary found in 15–20 percent of women. Women with polycystic ovarian syndrome may have other symptoms, which include a tendency to obesity, excessive body hair, and acne. The ovary seems to produce an excessive amount of male hormones. The condition may cause fertility problems and sufferers may have irregular periods.

What causes it?
The exact cause is not known. There may be a hormonal imbalance, but whether this is a cause or consequence of the syndrome remains to be worked out fully.

What might the doctor do?
Polycystic ovaries are often discovered because of one of the complaints listed above. The doctor will examine you internally and will probably arrange an ultrasound examination of your ovaries and blood tests to confirm the diagnosis. You may be given the oral contraceptive pill to stimulate a normal monthly period and combat the excessive male hormones. Fertility treatment could be necessary if you are having difficulties in conceiving.

What can I do?
Discuss the symptoms fully with your doctor so you understand the nature of all the treatments that are offered to you.

What is the outlook?
The outlook for women with polycystic ovaries depends on the severity of the problems encountered. Currently available treatments provide good control of the majority of symptoms.

WHAT HAPPENS DURING SURGERY?

• Benign ovarian cysts may be punctured and their contents carefully sucked out through the laparoscope.
• If the cyst is too large or if there is suspicion of a malignancy, the type of abdominal operation will depend on the appearance of the cyst and your age.
• In younger women, the benign cyst will be removed and the ovary conserved if possible. In older women with a benign cyst, the whole ovary will be removed. Women in their middle forties onward are usually offered the option to have both ovaries and their uterus removed.
• If both ovaries are removed you will be offered estrogen replacement therapy to prevent menopausal symptoms.

WHAT CAN I DO?

Discuss all of the possibilities with your doctor before you agree to have an operation. Ask her whether it will be absolutely necessary to have both ovaries removed and about taking ERT (estrogen replacement therapy).

WHAT IS THE OUTLOOK?

There is an excellent outlook for benign cysts. Even if it is necessary to remove both ovaries, the possibility of ERT means that you will have few of the problems associated with menopause.

SEE ALSO:
Hysterectomy, *page 79*
Laparoscopy, *page 77*
Menstrual Problems, *page 33*
Menopause, *page 18*
Ovarian Cancer, *page 44*
Pelvic Examination, *page 70*
Ultrasound Scan, *page 75*

OVARIAN CANCER

Rarely, ovarian cysts may be malignant. They tend to occur in childless women over the age of 35. Unfortunately, malignant cysts do not usually cause any symptoms until they have grown to a large size, by which time they may be very difficult to treat effectively.

WHAT CAUSES IT?

There are many theories about what causes malignant ovarian cysts to develop. They are more common in older women and in women who have not had children. They are less common in women who have used oral contraceptives and HRT for a number of years, and in those women who started their periods late and had an early menopause.

"Resting" the ovary – that is, periods in a woman's life when ovulation is suppressed, for example during pregnancy or while using oral contraceptives – may protect a woman against the development of ovarian cancer. Genetic factors have also been shown to be important in the development of ovarian cancer.

SYMPTOMS

- *Abdominal pain*
- *Swelling of the abdomen*
- *A hard lump in the abdomen*
- *If the cyst is large, pressure on the bladder can cause frequent urination*
- *Occasional breathlessness if the tumor puts pressure on the diaphragm*

SHOULD I SEE THE DOCTOR?

Some families carry a gene called BRCA1 that increases the likelihood of both ovarian and breast cancer. Genetic tests for this gene are now available to help identify those women at risk of developing ovarian and breast cancer.

If you have a history of ovarian or breast cancer in your family, it is important to tell your doctor.

WHAT MIGHT THE DOCTOR DO?

- Malignant cysts need more thorough surgery than benign ovarian cysts, depending on the type of tumor found. The doctor will attempt to remove the whole tumor and any deposits.
- Minimal surgery involves the removal of both ovaries and the fallopian tubes as well as the uterus.
- If the disease has already spread beyond the reproductive organs, much more extensive surgery will be necessary, involving the removal of other organs such as the bowel and bladder.
- Radiation therapy may also be used after surgery for malignant cysts.

WHAT IS THE OUTLOOK?

- If a malignancy is found, further treatment may well be necessary. Chemotherapy will be started to help shrink the tumor. Medicines containing platinum are commonly used to treat ovarian cancer, but radiation therapy alone has not been found to be effective for it.
- Further surgery may well be performed to find out if the chemotherapy has worked or to remove any recurrences.
- The outlook in the longer term depends on the stage of the disease and the type of malignant cell present in the ovary.

SEE ALSO:
Hysterectomy, *page 79*
Laparoscopy, *page 77*
Menstrual Problems, *page 33*
Ovarian Cysts, *page 42*
Ultrasound Scan, *page 75*

UTERINE CANCER

This rare cancer results from a malignant growth in the lining of the uterus, the endometrium. It is sometimes known as endometrial cancer. Cervical cancer can also sometimes be referred to as uterine cancer because the cervix is part of the uterus. Precancerous forms of the disease may exist for many years before the condition becomes malignant.

This cancer is more common in older women (less than 5 percent of sufferers are under 40), in those who used DES during pregnancy (or whose mothers did), and in those of higher socioeconomic groups. There has been a lot of controversy during recent years about the incidence of uterine cancer among women who take estrogen replacement therapy (ERT) for menopausal symptoms. If ERT is used, a menstrual period is usually induced every three months by a 14-day course of progestogen or the insertion of a progesterone IUD.

SYMPTOMS
- *Abnormal vaginal bleeding, between menstrual periods or after intercourse*
- *Heavy or prolonged menstrual periods*
- *Postmenopausal bleeding*
- *Cramping pain in the lower abdomen*
- *Pressure in the lower abdomen*
- *Frequency of urination due to pressure of the tumor on the bladder*

SHOULD I SEE THE DOCTOR?

If you have any change in your normal menstrual pattern or if you have any post-menopausal vaginal bleeding, consult your doctor immediately.

WHAT MIGHT THE DOCTOR DO ?

- If your doctor suspects that you have a growth in your uterus, the only effective way to check whether there is any malignancy is to undergo a **D&C** (dilatation and curettage) investigation.

- If the uterine lining has some cancerous cells, your doctor will recommend a total hysterectomy with removal of the ovaries and fallopian tubes as well as the uterus. This is nearly always combined with four to six weeks of radiation therapy.
- If the growth is advanced, an extended total **hysterectomy** will be performed to remove the top of the vagina and the glands of the pelvis too.

WHAT IS THE OUTLOOK?

The news is good. The overall cure rate is as high as 90 percent when the cancer is localized to the lining of the uterus itself. If the spread is beyond the lining and the muscles of the uterus, the figure after five years is reduced to a 40 percent cure rate.

SEE ALSO:
Abnormal Bleeding, *page 36*
Cervical Cancer, *page 26*
D&C, *page 82*
Fibroids, *page 41*
Hysterectomy, *page 79*
Hysteroscopy, *page 74*
Menstrual Problems, *page 33*

PELVIC INFLAMMATORY DISEASE

This is a general term used to describe grumbling inflammation of any of the pelvic organs: the uterus, fallopian tubes, or ovaries. Irrevocable scarring of the fallopian tubes and ovaries is the most serious complication because it causes sterility. Others include scarring and **painful intercourse** (dyspareunia). At one time, the most common cause of this disease was tuberculosis. Now it is **chlamydia**. There is some evidence that the use of intrauterine contraceptive devices may be a contributing factor.

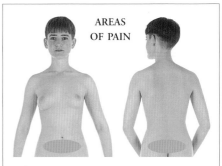

AREAS
OF PAIN

Pelvic pain
The most common symptoms of PID are abdominal pain and backache, both of which can cause acute discomfort.

SYMPTOMS
- *Abdominal pain*
- *Back pain*
- *Persistent menstrual-like cramps*
- *Vaginal spotting of blood*
- *Fatigue*
- *Pain during and after intercourse*
- *Foul-smelling vaginal discharge*
- *Flu-type symptoms of fever and chills*
- *Subfertility or infertility*

SHOULD I SEE THE DOCTOR?

PID must be treated early to prevent long-term problems. The symptoms can be those of an acute infection with fever, nausea, discomfort, and pain, which should alert you to the fact that there is something wrong. A chronic infection may cause only recurrent mild pain and sometimes backache. But both forms must be investigated. Don't wait for it to go away; see your doctor as soon as possible. If you have an IUD, go to your clinic immediately.

WHAT MIGHT THE DOCTOR DO?

- You will be examined and tested to identify the organism causing the infection. Your doctor will probably prescribe antibiotics and bed rest. Eat well and don't have sexual intercourse during the course of treatment. If antibiotics are not suitable for you, you may have to have more treatment.

- If PID develops into a chronic infection, it can be difficult to eradicate. You may need investigative laparoscopy to confirm the diagnosis. In severe cases, for a long-term infection, **hysterectomy** may be the only course of action, although you should go through any alternatives fully before agreeing to this operation.

WHAT CAN I DO?

- Don't let any vaginal discharge continue for any length of time without full investigation and treatment. Since PID can recur, have a full checkup to confirm that your infection has been completely eradicated.
- If you suspect that you or your partner may have a venereal disease, go to a sexually transmitted diseases clinic right away.

SEE ALSO:
Chlamydia, *page 54*
Contraception, *page 14*
Ectopic Pregnancy, *page 68*
Fertility Problems, *page 59*
Hysterectomy, *page 79*
Laparoscopy, *page 77*
Miscarriage, *page 71*
Painful Intercourse, *page 48*

SEXUAL
PROBLEMS

A fulfilling sex life should be a basic part of
human existence. For some people, however,
things aren't that simple at least some of the time,
because various problems occur that prevent them
from enjoying their relationships to the full.
Basic complaints, such as painful intercourse,
lack of sex drive, and vaginismus (vaginal spasms
that can prevent intercourse) are described here,
with the emphasis on what can be done to
cure or alleviate them, so that your lovemaking
can improve or resume.

PAINFUL INTERCOURSE

Any type of pain or discomfort during sexual intercourse, whether because of a local genital problem or pain deep in the pelvis is known as dyspareunia. It can vary from mild discomfort or tightness to an extreme pain that prevents intercourse altogether. Psychological factors are by far the most common cause. Inhibitions about the sexual act, resentment, anger, fear, or shame – and anticipating that sex will be unsuccessful – are all causes of disturbed psychological attitudes affecting sex.

SYMPTOMS
- *Pain during intercourse; either externally or deep in the pelvis during penetration*
- *Lack of desire or inclination for sex*
- *Involuntary closing of the legs and vagina to prevent penetration (vaginismus)*
- *Dryness in the vagina*

ARE THERE PHYSICAL REASONS?

There are several medical conditions that must be eliminated first. These include vaginal infections, PID (**pelvic inflammatory disease**), **endometriosis**, **prolapsed uterus**, urinary tract infection, irritation of the vulva (**pruritis vulvae**), hormonal deficiency at **menopause** or after childbirth causing dryness in the vagina, and painful perineal scars after an episiotomy.

SHOULD I SEE THE DOCTOR?

If you experience physical pain during intercourse or for some reason you are reluctant to permit your partner to penetrate your vagina, see your doctor.

WHAT MIGHT THE DOCTOR DO?

- Your doctor will examine you to check for any underlying disorder. If you have an infection, antibiotics should clear it up. If the discomfort is the result of poor stitching

after childbirth, your doctor may advise you to wait another couple of weeks, or to have the area restitched. This depends on how recently you have given birth.
- If your problem is not a physical one, your doctor will refer you to a sexual counselor, who will try to uncover the reasons for your fear of sexual intercourse. However, if your relationship is no longer a loving one, sex counseling will not help. It is not possible to heal a broken relationship with sex and you and your partner should admit this from the outset.

WHAT CAN I DO?

- Don't keep quiet about your expectations and preferences. You have to take responsibility for your own pleasure. Try to discuss this with your partner and try not to feel guilty about ordinary sexual practices. The only prerequisite for good sex is loving your partner, and if you do, most of your sexual problems should be resolved.
- If your problem has a physical cause, find other ways of showing affection.
- Forget labels. No woman is frigid. If you label yourself or are labeled frigid, you may become anxious and lose hope.
- Remember also that even if you are aroused by your partner, unless you have sufficient clitoral stimulation and your vagina lubricates sufficiently to make penetration easy and comfortable, you won't experience good sex. You may find you need to use a lubricating jelly.

SEE ALSO:
Cystitis, *page 28*
Endometriosis, *page 40*
Menopause, *page 18*
Pelvic Inflammatory Disease, *page 46*
Prolapse, *page 30*
Pruritis Vulvae, *page 22*
Vaginismus, *page 50*

LACK OF SEX DRIVE

Problems with intercourse and lack of interest can stem from both physical and emotional factors. It can become a chronic problem and failure to discuss it will have an effect on your relationships, and your image of yourself as a woman.

WHAT CAUSES IT?

Physical causes of lack of desire include diabetes, pain during intercourse, taking certain drugs such as alcohol or barbiturates, or taking an oral contraceptive that is high in estrogens. Removal of the ovaries (as part of a **hysterectomy)** depletes the supply of testosterone, which is believed to be the hormone that affects libido. An underactive thyroid gland reduces energy and sex drive.

Some of the symptoms that make sex uncomfortable and painful relate to sexually transmitted diseases, so ask your partner whether he has had intercourse with anyone else recently.

Fear is the most common cause of loss of desire. A woman may be fearful of letting herself go both physically and emotionally. She may have ambivalent feelings about intercourse, stemming from some incident in early life. These feelings will inevitably be transferred onto her partners. She may use her reluctance to punish herself; wanting to enjoy sex but hating herself for doing so. She may be angry with her partner or lovemaking may be rather predictable. Pregnancy is often a fear if **contraception** isn't discussed and practiced.

WHAT CAN I DO?

• Professional counseling is often the answer, particularly if there is friction in a relationship. A sexual counselor will try to uncover the reasons for your fear, although if your relationship is no longer a loving one, sex counseling will not help. A broken relationship cannot be helped with sex and this needs to be admitted by both partners at the outset of any therapy.

• Many women prefer to attend sex clinics where women are treated on their own by counseling, followed by masturbation training. The view is that a woman must be able to excite herself before she can be excited by anyone else.

• Sexual counseling is normally carried out at a special clinic, where trained counselors conduct physical and psychological tests. The types of problems that would be dealt with by a counselor are nearly always looked upon as something couples have to explore together, requiring frank discussion.

• If you feel that sexual counseling will be useful for you, the first step you have to take is to admit that you have a problem, and this will mean you have to overcome many inhibitions.

WHAT MIGHT THE COUNSELOR DO?

• Depending on the particular problem, you will be given advice about relaxing and losing your anxieties. The counselor will encourage you to go back to the beginning and find out how your body responds to sexual contact.

• She will suggest that you return to the simplest exploration of your partner's body through touch without sexual response. She will also teach you to concentrate on feelings and experiences, but to forget about orgasm for the time being.

• She will ask you to refrain from sexual intercourse for a few days or weeks.

• Later she will advise you to go on to enjoy touching, fondling, and caressing each other, then to orgasm without intercourse, and finally to orgasm during intercourse.

SEE ALSO:

Contraception, *page 14*
Menopause, *page 18*
Pruritis Vulvae, *page 22*

VAGINISMUS

This is an involuntary spasm of the muscles around the entrance to the vagina, causing the opening almost to close whenever an attempt is made to insert something, such as a speculum, tampon, or penis, into the vagina. The spasm can be so great that it prevents intercourse or makes penetration extremely painful. Sexual drive and arousal are usually normal until penetration itself is attempted. The pelvic floor muscles then tighten up, virtually closing the vaginal entrance, and a sufferer will arch her back and close her legs.

SYMPTOMS
- *Intense pain and difficulty during intercourse*
- *Involuntary closing of the vagina; the thighs often close tightly too*
- *Acute fear of penetration of any kind*

WHAT CAUSES IT?

Vaginismus usually occurs in anxiety-prone individuals who have never been able to insert a tampon or a finger into the vagina because of the anticipation that this will be painful. In some women, a contributing factor may be underlying guilt or fear associated with the sexual act, due to a restrictive upbringing or an inadequate sex education. Vaginismus can also occur when a woman is in sexual disharmony with her partner. Disharmony is often the result of a partner liking the idea of something that the other is repelled by. There can also be difficulty if the role a woman wants to play – active or passive – is at odds with her partner's likes and dislikes. Vaginismus may also result after a traumatic experience, such as rape.

SHOULD I SEE THE DOCTOR?

If you find you are unable to enjoy sex, see your doctor and talk it over. Don't let it fester because it may cause disenchantment with intercourse altogether.

WHAT MIGHT THE DOCTOR DO?

- Your doctor will first of all examine you to rule out the possibility of any anatomical abnormalities that could cause pain that results in spasm.
- He may then put you in touch with a sexual counselor or marriage guidance clinic where counseling for this kind of problem is undertaken. You may also like to make contact with a self-help group.
- Many women who experience vaginismus are not familiar with their sex organs. Some therapists work by helping you familiarize yourself with your genitalia. By learning that the insertion of your own finger or a speculum into your vagina is not painful, you may gain confidence about allowing penetration by your partner's penis.

WHAT CAN I DO?

- Vaginismus is an uncommon result of sexual problems but be reassured, most problems don't stem from you or your inadequacy. You are not abnormal.
- Look at your sexual relationship, see where the disharmony lies, and discuss it with your partner. The most common problem is when you feel something is distasteful. Perhaps oral sex, anal intercourse, or too frequent lovemaking upsets you.
- Talk about your likes and dislikes with your partner. If he understands, you should both acknowledge that neither of you is abnormal for wanting it, or for not wanting it, and that it is not selfish to refuse, although it is selfish to insist on something that either partner finds distasteful.

SEE ALSO:
Painful Intercourse, *page 48*
Pruritis Vulvae, *page 22*

SEXUALLY TRANSMITTED DISEASES

It can be distressing to realize that you might be suffering from an infection passed on by a partner, even when that infection is relatively minor, such as genital herpes or warts. There are, unfortunately, also more serious problems that can be transmitted sexually and which need urgent treatment. These range from the serious, such as gonorrhea, to the terrifying, such as AIDS. In the following pages, each complaint is described in detail to help recognition, and the various treatment options available are outlined.

GENITAL HERPES

This is a common viral disease transmitted during sexual intercourse when the virus is active in the surface layers of the skin around the genitals. Millions of people are infected with the virus but probably only one quarter of them experience symptoms.

Herpes is caused by the *herpes simplex II* virus. The virus is transmitted through exposed raw areas of skin and is more common in women because their genital areas are warmer and more moist than men's. Herpes is highly contagious and there is a high chance of catching it if either partner has an active blister; it can also be caught from people who don't have symptoms. The symptoms appear between three and twenty days after sexual contact with an infected partner.

Today herpes is considered incurable but manageable; once in the body the virus stays there although treatment can clear the symptoms or suppress activity. The waxing and waning course of the disease can cause the sufferer much psychological misery as well as physical pain.

SYMPTOMS

- *For a primary attack, many women sufferers have no symptoms*
- *The skin on the vulva feels sensitive to the touch, ticklish, even numb*
- *Blisters appear within a few hours, enlarge, burst, and become painful ulcers within two or three days*
- *The ulcers form scabs and take 14–21 days to disappear*
- *Pain on urination*
- *There may be a raised temperature and swollen glands in the groin*

SHOULD I SEE THE DOCTOR?

See your doctor immediately if you feel numb or sensitive in the genital area, if blisters appear, or if you have had sexual relations with anyone with the herpes virus.

WHAT MIGHT THE DOCTOR DO?

- There is no cure for genital herpes but new oral antiviral treatments, if taken early enough, are often effective both in limiting the blisters and shortening the attack. Idoxuridine, in an ointment or liquid cream, is still successful for some.
- Other remedies include daily douches with providone iodine solution, or painting the blisters with gentian violet. Your doctor may also prescribe an antibiotic.
- It is possible to transmit the virus to a newborn baby during delivery. If you have an attack when your baby is due, your doctor may suggest a cesarean.

WHAT CAN I DO?

- A long soak in a tepid bath can help, as can cold packs applied directly to the labia and vulva. Do not use ice cubes.
- About 50 percent of herpes sufferers have another attack, so try to recognize the early warning signs and treat them at once.
- Irritation of the vagina from other causes is known to trigger attacks, so can stress, fever, cold, menstrual periods, and tight-fitting clothes.
- To avoid the virus do not have sex with someone who is infected, and do not have sex if you have the active disease. Condoms must always be worn for penetrative sex.
- Prevent recurrences with lots of rest and a balanced diet. Manage stress by learning relaxation exercises or yoga. Many sufferers feel unclean and stigmatized; try to overcome this feeling through counseling.
- Since there is a greater risk of **cervical cancer** in women who have had herpes, you must have regular **cervical smears**.

SEE ALSO:
Cervical Cancer, *page 26*
Cervical Smear, *page 71*
Genital Problems, *page 21*

GENITAL WARTS

Genital warts are the most common sexually transmitted disease. They are small, benign lumps of skin that appear on the vulva and anus, inside the vagina, and on the cervix.

WHAT CAUSES THEM?

Genital warts are caused by the same virus that causes warts on other parts of the body. The virus is called HPV or the *human papillomavirus*, and can be spread through personal and sexual contact. It is possible to transfer the virus from one part of the body to the genital region, although this is rare.

Genital warts are most often transmitted sexually. It may take several months after infection before a wart becomes visible in the genital region.

SYMPTOMS

- *A single raised, soft wart, or a group of warts, in and around the entrance of the vagina and the anus*
- *A cluster of tiny, itchy lumps on the perineal skin (the area between the genitals and the anus), on the labia, or inside the vagina, including right up to the cervix*

SHOULD I SEE THE DOCTOR?

Genital warts do not usually cause any discomfort. However, left untreated they may grow and spread. There is also the risk that they may be transmitted to a new sexual partner. Perhaps the most serious consequence of infection with HPV is the increased risk of developing **cervical cancer** that untreated infection brings. The diagnosis of genital warts is made on the basis of your doctor's examination.

WHAT MIGHT THE DOCTOR DO?

- Treatment of genital warts depends on their location. After examining you thoroughly and perhaps screening you for other sexually transmitted diseases, the doctor may prescribe a special lotion called podophyllin, which you will be asked to apply to the warts, carefully avoiding any surrounding healthy skin. If the warts are in a difficult location, it is sometimes best for medical staff to apply the lotion for you, to prevent damage to the surrounding skin.
- If podophyllin does not succeed in clearing the warts after a few weeks, stronger agents such as trichloroacetic acid could be used. Occasionally the genital warts may be frozen off with liquid nitrogen and, rarely, a laser may be used to burn them away.
- If you haven't had a **cervical smear** recently, your doctor will take one, and may arrange a **colposcopy** to make sure your cervix is free from infection.
- Apart from the increased risk of an abnormal smear test, there are very few other complications of infection with the HPV virus.

WHAT CAN I DO?

- As soon as you notice any abnormal area of skin in or around your genital area, it is best to see your doctor.
- Having a regular smear test will also protect you from the dangers of untreated infection with HPV by detecting the disease promptly. You must ask your doctor to explain all of the treatments she suggests to you.
- Try to persuade your sexual partner to see his doctor or attend a genitourinary clinic to check for genital warts.

SEE ALSO:
Cervical Cancer, *page 26*
Cervical Smear, *page 71*
Colposcopy, *page 72*

Chlamydia

Any sexually active woman runs the risk of getting chlamydia, especially if she has multiple partners. Women with untreated infections risk losing their fertility, hence the alarm now caused by this once little-known disorder. Although easy to treat, chlamydia is difficult to diagnose because symptoms are usually slow to develop, mild, or nonexistent. But as long as there is awareness of the possibility of the disease, modern tests and treatments can eradicate it before any serious consequences develop.

Theoretically, chlamydia infects the linings of the vagina, mouth, eyes, the urinary tract, or the rectum, but in women the infection is usually confined to the cervix, leading to an offensive yellow-colored discharge. About one third of cases can go on to **pelvic inflammatory disease**, which damages the fallopian tubes and causes infertility.

Chlamydia may also be responsible for **ectopic pregnancy**, which is potentially life-threatening. During childbirth an infected woman may infect her baby. Often, a pregnant woman with chlamydia will be recommended for a cesarean section.

Symptoms
- *Most women sufferers have no real symptoms*
- *Once it gains a hold, there can be unusual discharge*
- *Abdominal pain, particularly during sexual intercourse*
- *Fever*

Should I See the Doctor?

If you have any symptoms of unusual discharge or, more likely, your sexual partner has these symptoms, go to see your doctor as soon as possible, or go to the nearest sexually transmitted diseases clinic. It is very important to treat this disease as early as possible.

What Might the Doctor Do?

At one time it was necessary to take a specimen of the vaginal secretions in order to culture chlamydia in a laboratory. This entailed waiting at least 48 hours for the result of the tests. However, new laboratory tests have been devised that can give results in 30–60 minutes, thus permitting immediate treatment.

What is the Treatment?

- Chlamydia is simply and completely cured with a course of antibiotics. It is essential to take the medication exactly as prescribed and to complete the full course. Do not stop taking the pills because the symptoms disappear; the chlamydia could return. It is essential that your partner is treated at the same time.
- If the diagnosis is wrongly stated as **gonorrhea**, the treatment given will not cure the chlamydia. Therefore, since many people with gonorrhea also have chlamydia, and penicillin is not adequate, tetracyclines or sulfonamides are used.

What Can I Do?

- If you have many sexual contacts, all of them must be informed of the infection, and screened and treated if necessary.
- To prevent reinfection use barrier contraceptives such as condoms and diaphragms with spermicidal creams.

See also:
Contraception, *page 14*
Ectopic Pregnancy, *page 68*
Fertility Problems, *page 59*
Pelvic Inflammatory Disease, *page 46*
Vaginal Discharge, *page 23*

GONORRHEA

This is a common venereal disease that is caused by the bacterium *Neisseria gonorrhoeae*. It can affect both men and women, and in five out of every six women infected by the bacterium there are no symptoms, which makes it more dangerous. The most serious aspect of this disease is that if it remains untreated during the incubation period (usually between about two and ten days), it progresses to the chronic form that sets up inflammation in the pelvis. If the ovaries and fallopian tubes are affected, they may become blocked and the scarring may cause infertility.

The risk of contracting gonorrhea seems to become higher if you are using oral contraceptives – the infection seems to spread more quickly. The most common way many women suspect they may have become infected, is if they notice the recognizable symptoms of the disease in their male partners.

SYMPTOMS

- *There may be vaginal discharge with pain and a burning sensation when urinating*
- *The entire perineum (the area between the genitals and the anus) may be sore, and inflammation of the rectum causes pain when passing a stool*
- *A sore throat if the bacterium has been passed there during oral sex*
- *Penile discharge in your partner*

SHOULD I SEE THE DOCTOR?

If you suspect that you have gonorrhea, go to your doctor or to a sexually transmitted disease clinic and don't have any sexual contact with anyone until you are cured.

WHAT MIGHT THE DOCTOR DO?

- Diagnosis of gonorrhea can be difficult, so your doctor will take some samples of the secretions from your urethra, cervix, and rectum and send them to a laboratory for further investigation. There is no reliable blood test.
- Special STD clinics give the best results, so even if you have a negative test and you know or think you may have had intercourse with someone with gonorrhea, insist on more tests or treatment.

WHAT IS THE TREATMENT?

- Penicillin is the mainstay of treatment and may be given in a slow-release injectable form which requires only the one injection, making treatment easy. If the organism is resistant, ciprofloxacin can be given.
- You should then have a full gynecological examination to make sure the disease hasn't caused **pelvic inflammatory disease**. Have a repeat gonorrhea culture to ascertain that the infection is gone.
- Gonorrhea can mask the symptoms of other sexually transmitted diseases, so you should be tested for **syphilis** too.

WHAT CAN I DO?

- If you discover you have gonorrhea, give the clinic the names of your sexual contacts so that they can get treatment before they infect others. Stop all sexual activity until you have been cured.
- You would be wise to have an IUD removed. You can have a new one fitted when you are clear of infection.
- As with all sexually transmitted diseases, gonorrhea is most common among young people under the age of 25 who have many sexual partners. Using condoms will decrease the probability of getting an infection or being reinfected.
- Check that your partner is not a carrier, since he could reinfect you even after you have been successfully treated.

SEE ALSO:
Pelvic Inflammatory Disease, *page 46*
Syphilis, *page 56*

SYPHILIS

Two or three hundred years ago syphilis was the medical scourge of the time in very much the same way that **AIDS** is now. It is a venereal disease that infected large numbers of people of both sexes; even as recently as the 1930s, it was fatal for many.

With the discovery of penicillin, syphilis has been almost completely eradicated except in a few underdeveloped and underprivileged communities. Syphilis is caused by a bacterium, *Treponema pallidum*, and can be transmitted from person to person through sexual contact. There are four major stages of syphilis infection: primary, secondary, latent, and tertiary.

SYMPTOMS

- *For primary syphilis, a "chancre" or sore on the vulva and swollen glands in the groin*
- *For secondary syphilis, a rash, which can cover most of the body*
- *For tertiary syphilis, widespread problems, including blindness, brain damage, and paralysis*

SHOULD I SEE THE DOCTOR?

Primary and secondary syphilis can be treated and cured completely with a single course of penicillin. It is therefore a great tragedy if the disease goes undiagnosed. If you suspect that you may have contracted syphilis, seek confidential medical attention immediately. Unfortunately, once the disease has destroyed certain tissues, such as joints, it is impossible to cure.

WHAT MIGHT THE DOCTOR DO?

- The diagnosis will be made after a blood test and taking samples from the sore or rash. Treatment involves a course of antibiotic injections.
- You should have regular blood tests for at least two years after contracting syphilis to ensure that the disease has been cured.

WHAT CAN I DO?

- Avoid casual sexual contacts.
- If you discover a genital or any other kind of sore that you can't account for, have a medical checkup.
- If you suspect that you may have caught a venereal disease, go to your sexually transmitted diseases clinic for a blood test.
- You can help eradicate the disease if you give the names of all your sexual partners to your doctor or the clinic so they can be traced and treated. Because the disease can be cured, it is imperative that all partners are treated; otherwise, the risks remain. This information is always kept confidential.

SEE ALSO:
Chlamydia, *page 54*
Gonorrhea, *page 55*
HIV/AIDS, *page 57*

HIV/AIDS

Acquired immune deficiency syndrome is more commonly known as AIDS. It is caused by the human immunodeficiency virus (HIV). There are two types of HIV, type 1 and type 2; infection with either form can lead to AIDS, although HIV-2 seems to be a less aggressive form of the virus.

While HIV is infectious, it is not as contagious as some other viruses such as the common cold or influenza. It cannot, for example, be caught simply by touching and normal social contact, and is not spread by coughs and sneezes.

It is usually transmitted by the mixing of body fluids – mainly blood, semen, and vaginal secretions. The most common route of transmission is through sexual intercourse but it may also be passed on via blood transfusions and the sharing of needles by intravenous drug users.

The virus is also found in saliva and tears, although the concentration of viral particles is too low to be infectious. HIV affects all racial and social groups, as well as both heterosexuals and homosexuals.

AIDS weakens the body's natural immune system to such an extent that it is unable to fight off opportunistic infections or control cancerous growths. AIDS sufferers often succumb to diseases that rarely cause any illness in the general population.

SYMPTOMS

- *Marked weight loss over a relatively short period of time*
- *Enlarged lymph glands*
- *Many HIV sufferers have infections such as pneumonia, oral thrush, herpes simplex, or shingles*
- *Cancers, such as Kaposi's sarcoma and lymphoma, and opportunistic autoimmune diseases*
- *Dementia-like syndrome when brain and nervous system are affected*

HOW CAN I TELL IF I AM HIV POSITIVE?

The body's response to infection with HIV is to produce antibodies, although they may take up to three months to appear. You would only be identified as HIV positive when antibodies are detected in your blood. For that reason, if you take an AIDS test too soon after possible exposure, it can be negative. It is usually recommended that you take a test about six months after you suspect infection may have taken place.

An HIV-positive person does not necessarily have AIDS, which may take up to ten years to develop, during which time he or she may remain well. It is therefore possible for people to be unaware they are HIV positive and to pass on the virus unknowingly.

WHERE DID HIV COME FROM?

There are many theories about how the virus first entered the human population. HIV probably arose as a variant of a virus affecting African monkeys and apes. It was able to cross over to infect the human population of Africa, from where it spread to the rest of the world. Although it originally affected the homosexual community in the West, heterosexual transmission is now the main form of transmission worldwide.

HOW CAN I PREVENT IT?

- The main route of HIV infection is through sex. It may be passed through both vaginal and anal intercourse. Sexual transmission may be prevented, however, by the use of good-quality condoms. Spermicides actually kill the AIDS virus so they must always be used.
- Theoretically, sexual intercourse with only one infected individual is enough to pass on the HIV virus. Since it is impossible to tell whether an individual is HIV positive from his or her appearance, precautions must be used with all new sexual partners.

HIV/AIDS: CONTINUED

• Intravenous drug users can pass on the virus by sharing needles and syringes, so sharing needles should always be avoided.

• HIV has also been transmitted through infected blood products; the major group to be infected in this way were hemophiliacs. Now, however, all blood products are screened for HIV in most developed countries.

• Transmission from an HIV-positive mother to her baby may also occur during pregnancy, birth, or breast-feeding.

WOMEN AND HIV

Women need to be assertive in order to protect themselves from HIV. The practice of "safe sex" should be compulsory for everyone until such time as you are able to confirm that your partner is HIV negative. Since it can take up to three months to produce antibodies, it's best to practice safe sex until this "window of infection" is passed, and it should only be relaxed if your partner

TESTING FOR HIV

The usual test for HIV infection involves analyzing a blood sample for signs of HIV antibodies. (Antibodies are substances produced by the body to fight off infection by a particular virus.) The presence of antibodies in your blood, therefore, indicates that there is an infection from the virus present. This is why anyone whose blood tests positive for HIV antibodies is said to be HIV positive. The HIV virus incubates for a period of several months before becoming active, so there is a gap between exposure to the virus and evidence that infection has developed. For that reason, if you take an AIDS test too soon after possible exposure it can be negative. It is usually recommended that you take a test about six months after you suspect infection may have taken place.

does not engage in any other potential high-risk activity such as intravenous drug use or unprotected intercourse with another person.

WHAT IS THE TREATMENT?

• Following a diagnosis of HIV, treatment is begun to try to slow down the rate of viral replication. Various drugs are prescribed to achieve this aim, and different combinations are being researched and developed all the time.

• These treatments have side effects but they do seem to decrease the rate of HIV multiplication in the body.

• Treatment of opportunistic infections depends on the specific agent infecting the patient. High-dose antibiotics and antiviral drugs are often given routinely to prevent an infection from taking hold.

CAN HIV/AIDS BE CURED?

Although the progression of HIV infection to AIDS may be slowed down, there is still no cure for AIDS, nor is there a vaccine to prevent infection with HIV. The problem is compounded because HIV attacks the immune system – the route by which the body is usually able to fight infections and cancers. HIV-1 and 2 also seem to consist of various subtypes, which makes the likelihood of finding a universal vaccine remote.

Death is nearly always due to overwhelming pneumonia or Kaposi's sarcoma. The brain may be affected terminally giving rise to an illness resembling dementia.

SEE ALSO:
Contraception, *page 14*
Genital Herpes, *page 52*
Thrush, *page 24*

CHAPTER 7

FERTILITY PROBLEMS

Becoming pregnant is usually one of the great joys
of life; failure to become pregnant can therefore
be traumatic. In the pages that follow,
both physical and emotional reasons for problems
such as infertility, miscarriage, and ectopic pregnancy
are discussed in detail. Possible solutions, such
as surgery, hormone treatment, and assisted
conception, are also explored. The accent is
on the positive and practical ways to cope
with the problem and the many effective
solutions now available.

PROBLEMS WITH FERTILITY

Infertility means the inability to conceive. Very few women and couples are truly infertile; a much higher number are sub-fertile – in other words, they have difficulty in conceiving. About one in ten couples have some period of subfertility in their lives. The fertility of a couple is the sum of both of their fertilities, and infertility must therefore be investigated with the cooperation of both partners.

WHAT CAUSES INFERTILITY?

In about 40 percent of infertile couples, the problem lies with the man. About 40 percent of cases are due to problems in the woman, and the remainder are due to shared problems of one sort or another.

Male problems
Male problems include the complete inability of the testes to produce sperm (fortunately very rare); low sperm count due to an abnormality of the testes; a larger than normal number of abnormal sperm; and impotence, premature ejaculation, or inability to sustain an erection.

Female problems
• Failure to ovulate (release an egg) is the most common cause of female infertility, accounting for about one third of all infertile women.
• It may result from imbalances of the hormones that trigger ovulation, or from damage to the ovary from infection, surgery, or radiation treatment.

Mutual support
It is important to discuss fertility problems, treatments, and fears together, and to comfort and help each other, as you try to find out what the future holds.

Hormones may interfere with conception in other ways, not just by influencing ovulation. For example, progesterone is needed for a fertilized egg to survive – so the egg would be affected if too little is produced, or for too short a time.
• Healthy female reproductive organs are also essential for conception to occur naturally. Problems with the uterus account for at least ten percent of infertility cases. The uterus may be congenitally abnormal, or contain adhesions (bands of scars), polyps, or **fibroids**, or it may be affected by **endometriosis**.
• The fallopian tubes are the pathways that permit the ascending sperm to reach the egg and then allow the developing embryo to reach the uterus for implantation. An **ectopic pregnancy, pelvic inflammatory**

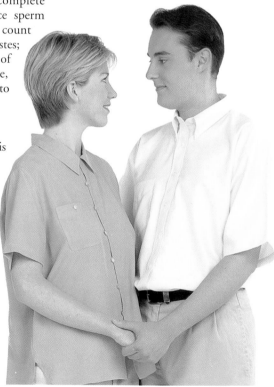

disease, surgical procedures, or even an infection of any kind (including sexually transmitted infections) could cause a blockage in the tubes or scarring that would prevent you from conceiving naturally.

• In order to reach an egg to fertilize it, sperm must swim through a large quantity of mucus secreted by the cervix. If the mucus is so thick that the sperm cannot penetrate it, or if it contains antibodies that attack the sperm directly, the sperm will never reach the egg and fertilization cannot therefore occur.

• Age is also a consideration. Around the age of 25, fertility begins to slowly diminish and after the age of 45 only half a woman's cycles are ovulatory. A woman over 45, therefore, has only half as many fertile periods annually as a younger woman.

Shared problems

Between 20 and 30 percent of fertility problems are "shared," usually because of what is called subfertility. Subfertility occurs when a woman's fertility is marginal, such as when she ovulates infrequently. Usually this only becomes a problem if her partner's fertility is also marginal – if he has a low to average sperm count, for instance – because subfertility in one partner can be balanced by strong fertility in the other.

SHOULD I SEE THE DOCTOR?

Whatever your age, if you've been having unprotected sex twice a week for at least a year, and you haven't become pregnant, consult your doctor. However, since some forms of treatment can take several years to complete (see overleaf), you may find that if you are over 35 it is worth consulting your doctor after about six to eight months of unprotected sexual intercourse and failure to conceive.

WHAT MIGHT THE DOCTOR DO?

• Your doctor will question you closely about your menstrual history, and you may be asked for the dates of your last six periods. He will also ask you how long you have been trying to have a baby, when you stopped using contraception, and about your family's medical history.

• You'll be asked about your own medical history, including any surgical operations or illnesses that could have a bearing on your fertility, such as anorexia nervosa; and to give details about any specific gynecological problems you may have experienced, such as **terminations of pregnancy** or sexually transmitted diseases.

• Both you and your partner will also be asked about your frequency of sexual intercourse. Although this may seem too obvious, your doctor will want to rule out the possibility that you are simply not having unprotected intercourse frequently enough to enable conception to occur. There may also be some psychological difficulties that need to be addressed, and the doctor may therefore refer you to a sexual counselor.

• You will then be given a physical examination to check the condition of your reproductive organs and your health in general. The precise examination will depend on your medical history and may involve your doctor looking into your eyes to check the retina or feeling your neck for any differences in your thyroid gland. Your breasts may also be examined to check for normal development.

• Your partner will also be asked about his medical and family history. The doctor will want to know, for example, if his testes did not descend in the normal way. He may also be questioned about his work environment, since environmental factors can sometimes result in a low sperm count. Childhood illnesses, such as mumps, and sexually transmitted diseases are also relevant. The doctor may then examine him to see if there is any obvious physical reason for infertility.

• You and your partner must be honest and thorough in your answers. Investigation of infertility can take a long time and be very

PROBLEMS WITH FERTILITY: CONTINUED

frustrating and sometimes embarrassing. If you are prepared for this, the strain will be easier to bear. While these investigations have been known to cause irreparable damage to a relationship, other couples find that they are brought closer together by the shared experience and their determination to become parents.

• This first examination will help the doctor determine which initial investigations and tests should be carried out. If you are an older woman wanting a first baby, ask for the program to be speeded up if at all possible because it takes time, and the doctor will optimize the treatment schedule if he can, although different centers have different policies about this.

WHAT TESTS ARE DONE?

• If your doctor suspects that some anatomical obstruction is causing the problem, basic tests will be carried out immediately. If, however, there seems to be no immediate and obvious reason for your inability to conceive, your doctor will first ask your partner to produce a sample of semen for analysis; there wouldn't be much point in carrying on with the various female tests if your partner is found to be infertile. The semen analysis will count the number of sperm, their motility (ability to move), and the number of abnormal sperm.

• The first step in investigating your infertility is to determine whether or not you are ovulating. Your doctor will therefore show you how to put together a basal body temperature (BBT) chart covering a period of three months. This will show whether or not your body temperature rises during the time of ovulation.

• You may also be given a progesterone blood test. If around the middle of your menstrual cycle your blood level contains the normal amount of progesterone, it is assumed that you are ovulating.

• Once the semen analysis and preliminary tests have been completed, it should be clear whether it is you or your partner who needs treatment.

WHAT IS THE TREATMENT?

• Actual treatment, of course, depends on what is thought to be the cause of the infertility, but your doctor is likely to refer you to a special fertility clinic for further investigation and help.

• The clinic can employ a whole battery of tests to help discover why you have been unable to conceive, including **ultrasound scanning** of the ovaries to confirm that ovulation is occurring, and **laparoscopy** to determine whether the fallopian tubes are damaged or blocked, and also to view the uterus for signs of problems that could prevent pregnancy, such as **endometriosis**, **fibroids**, or malformations.

• Once the problem has been diagnosed, treatment can usually proceed. This may be by surgery, fertility medications, or assisted conception techniques.

BLOCKED FALLOPIAN TUBES

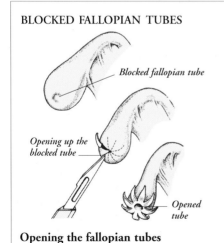

Blocked fallopian tube

Opening up the blocked tube

Opened tube

Opening the fallopian tubes
If fallopian tubes are blocked (top), they can be opened up (center) with micro-surgery. This enables the opened tube to carry sperm to the egg to fertilize it.

SURGICAL TECHNIQUES

• Blocked fallopian tubes may be opened with a microsurgical technique known as salpingostomy. **Ovarian cysts** and fibroids can also be removed surgically.

• Other surgical procedures may also have to be considered if you have miscarried recurrently and are unable to carry a baby to term. Abnormalities in the shape of the uterus and an incompetent cervix are two reasons for this problem.

FERTILITY DRUGS

• Fertility drugs are used when a hormone defect has been diagnosed. Specific therapy will be tailored according to your particular needs and often involves more than one drug. The risk of multiple pregnancy is increased and other side effects of this treatment may include headaches, hot flushes, and abdominal pain because the ovaries are enlarged.

• You may be given Clomiphene, which creates a menstrual period then encourages the pituitary gland to secrete estrogen so that the ovaries produce an egg. All through this therapy, during which the medicines are only administered for short periods of time during the cycle, your doctor will check your ovaries with an ultrasound scan to see if ovulation is occurring.

• If this treatment does not succeed in stimulating the ovaries, a daily injection of HMG (human menopausal gonadotropin) may be given to encourage the ovary to release an egg.

ASSISTED CONCEPTION

• Many childless couples have been helped by techniques to assist conception. These include sperm or egg donation and in vitro fertilization (IVF). However, the emotional costs of these treatments can be high, and it is essential that all the issues involved are discussed thoroughly before you proceed. Counseling for couples is provided by fertility clinics and hospitals.

ISSUES TO CONSIDER

There are a number of issues you need to resolve before embarking on what can be an emotional and long-lasting attempt to become pregnant.

• If you were to have a child using donor sperm or eggs, or both, would the fact that the child wasn't "yours" genetically prevent you from loving him or her as your own?

• Would you feel jealous if a donor's sperm or eggs were used to conceive a child with your partner?

• Would you tell your child how he or she was conceived, or would you try to keep it a secret?

• If you intend to keep it a secret, can you be sure that the truth won't come out, perhaps destructively, during a time of crisis?

• If your child was conceived by the use of donor sperm or eggs, how would you cope if your child wanted to trace his or her genetic parent in later life?

• How long would you persist with infertility treatment?

• What would you do with frozen sperm, eggs, or embryos that you do not use?

• Could you cope with a multiple pregnancy? What if one, some, or all of the babies died?

• You should also be aware that in vitro fertilization is very time-consuming. Even when you are eventually accepted for IVF, your treatment may then be delayed by a further year or more. This means that it could be four years from referral to receiving treament, which can be a long time to wait if you have postponed having a family until your mid- to late thirties.

SPERM DONATION

The most straightforward type of assisted conception is the artificial insemination of a woman with her partner's or a donor's

PROBLEMS WITH FERTILITY: CONTINUED

sperm. Donors are often university or medical students, and hospitals and clinics take great care to ensure that potential donors are in good physical and mental health, and have no known inheritable disorders in their family. Donors are always tested for HIV. They also try to make sure that your donor has similar physical characteristics to those of your partner.

• All information about the donor is strictly confidential. There is no mention of sperm donation in your maternity records, and your joint names can be given on the baby's birth certificate.

• Before you are inseminated, the clinic will have ascertained that you are ovulating using basal body temperature (BBT) charts or a luteinizing hormone (LH) predictor kit. An ultrasound scan just before ovulation can detect follicle growth and, if necessary, you will be given hormones to stimulate ovulation. The donor's sperm is then introduced into your cervical canal or uterus using a syringe.

• Donor insemination can seem to be the ideal solution for many infertile couples, but there are a number of points that should be carefully considered before going ahead, and good counseling is essential. First and foremost, the feelings of your partner need to be considered. It is not uncommon, for instance, for men to feel inadequate or jealous when a donor's sperm is used to impregnate their partners. In addition, some women are very repelled by the circumstances in which they conceive or by the fact that a different man's sperm can be used at each visit.

EGG DONATION

If a woman is unable to produce an egg of her own, those of a donor may be used instead. The egg is fertilized with your partner's sperm by in vitro fertilization (see right). This has the advantage that both of you are involved in the process: your partner fertilizes the egg and you will carry and give birth to the baby. However, it is a much more complicated procedure than sperm donation.

IN VITRO FERTILIZATION

Since the first test-tube baby was successfully delivered in 1978, tens of thousands of babies have been born by what is called in vitro fertilization (IVF). *In vitro* simply means "in glass," and refers to the glass dish in which sperm and eggs are combined in the laboratory. IVF involves the removal of eggs from the ovaries, fertilization with sperm in the laboratory, and transferral of the early embryos into the uterus. The process is as follows:

• First, a test is carried out to ensure that the sperm count is healthy. Then the eggs are collected. Most women only produce one egg per cycle, but because IVF needs several eggs, the ovaries are stimulated to produce more. This involves suppressing the woman's normal cycle, then stimulating the ovaries with special hormone injections so that they produce a number of eggs simultaneously. Over the next week or so, you will make several visits to the clinic so that the development of the eggs can be carefully monitored.

• To collect the eggs, a gynecologist will use ultrasound to give a clear picture of the reproductive tract. He or she will guide a thin, hollow probe in through the vagina and toward the ovary. Eggs are drawn into the probe by a gentle suction action. The probe is then withdrawn and the eggs are incubated for 24 hours.

• Once the eggs are fully mature, they are carefully placed in a culture medium with 100,000–200,000 sperm from your partner or donor for about 12–15 hours to allow fertilization to take place.

• Alternatively, a single sperm is carefully injected into the center of the egg through a glass pipette only one-tenth the width of a human hair. This technique is commonly known as ICSI (intracytoplasmic sperm injection).

• After two or three days in an incubator, a maximum of three of the best embryos are then transferred into your uterus. To minimize the risk of having twins, triplets, or even more multiple births, many fertility centers suggest implanting no more than two embryos at a time.

OTHER TECHNIQUES

Some fertility specialists use a number of other techniques to try to bring about a successful pregnancy.

• One such is GIFT (gamete intrafallopian tube transfer). Rather than fertilizing the egg in the laboratory, in this method the sperm and egg are transferred together into the open end of a fallopian tube, which thereby allows fertilization to occur naturally. The resulting embryo can then arrive in the uterus at the correct point in the cycle, allowing implantation to occur. The essential requirement for this procedure

is that at least one of your fallopian tubes must be healthy, and the drawback is that you have no idea whether fertilization has occurred, let alone implantation.

• One week after the day of egg retrieval, a blood sample is taken so that your progesterone level can be measured. If you have not had a menstrual period by about 16 days after retrieval, a test is then done to detect the pregnancy hormone beta-HCG. Finding the hormone present confirms to your doctor that at least one of the embryos has implanted successfully.

• The actual number of implanted embryos can be ascertained as early as 28 days after implantation, by using ultrasound.

WHAT IS THE OUTLOOK?

Only about ten percent of couples achieve pregnancy on the first attempt at in vitro fertilization and the overall success rate, leading to the birth of a healthy baby, is about 12–14 percent. With repeated IVF cycles, however, the pregnancy rate rises considerably to exceed 50 percent.

SEE ALSO:

Ectopic Pregnancy, *page 68*
Endometriosis, *page 40*
Fibroids, *page 41*
Laparoscopy, *page 77*
Ovarian Cysts, *page 42*
Pelvic Inflammatory Disease, *page 46*
Sexual Problems, *page 47*
Termination of Pregnancy, *page 85*
Ultrasound Scan, *page 75*

MISCARRIAGE

Sometimes called spontaneous abortion, this refers to the loss of a fetus before 24 weeks of pregnancy. The use of the word "abortion" sometimes leads to misunderstanding, but doctors use it to describe any pregnancy that ends suddenly, whether artificially or from natural causes.

Spontaneous abortions are much more common than is generally thought. Many miscarriages go undetected and many more go unreported. In fact, up to one third of all first pregnancies miscarry. Excluding unrecognized miscarriages, spontaneous miscarriage occurs in about 15 percent of all conceptions. There is usually a very good reason why a miscarriage occurs during the first trimester of a pregnancy.

SYMPTOMS
- *Bleeding from the vagina, either spotting or heavier*
- *Mucus in blood that has leaked from the vagina*
- *Backache and/or abdominal cramps*
- *Disappearance of the signs of pregnancy*

WHAT CAUSES IT?

A spontaneous abortion can result because of parental, fetal, or combined factors. These include:
- Defect in the egg or sperm resulting in an abnormal fetus.
- Abnormally shaped uterus which cannot sustain a pregnancy because of some anatomical problem.
- Uterine **fibroids**.
- Incompetent cervix in which the cervix opens rather than remains closed until labor begins; this is often the result of an unskilled induced abortion or a previous rapid labor.
- Placental insufficiency; the placenta fails or does not develop properly and so cannot nourish the fetus.

- Uncontrolled diabetes or very severe high blood pressure.
- Rhesus incompatibility.
- Maternal infections – bacterial or viral such as **syphilis** or rubella.

SHOULD I SEE THE DOCTOR?

If you know you are pregnant, or think you might be, and experience any vaginal bleeding and/or cramping pain at any time, call your doctor immediately.

While you are waiting for your doctor, go to bed and keep your feet raised. Wear a sanitary napkin if necessary. Do not flush away any of the discharge because your doctor will want to examine it.

WHAT MIGHT THE DOCTOR DO?

- With a threatened abortion, you will be advised to go to bed for 24 hours to wait and see – bed rest helps by increasing the flow of blood to the uterus.
- Low hormonal levels usually lead to a miscarriage; you will be advised to rest, although unfortunately it probably won't make any difference to the outcome.
- An **ultrasound scan** will determine whether the fetus is still alive or not, or whether there is any tissue left inside your uterus. In some cases of miscarriage there may be heavy blood loss, necessitating a blood transfusion.

WHAT IS THE SURGICAL TREATMENT?

- If some products of conception remain after an incomplete abortion (see panel, opposite), you will need to be admitted to hospital for an ERPC to remove it. (ERPC stands for "evacuation of the retained products of conception.")
- If there is a "missed abortion," the fetus will have to be removed surgically or by an induced labor. If you miscarry several times, you will have tests to try to find the specific cause.

• You may be given a **hysterosalpingogram** to check out the condition of your uterus and fallopian tubes.

• Your doctor will examine the aborted fetus and placenta as well in order to treat you appropriately. In some cases, you may be referred to an infertility expert.

• If you have a septic abortion, which means that your internal organs have become infected, you will be given antibiotics in large doses to combat infection, which is the most frequent cause of maternal death following abortion.

• An ERPC will be essential to remove the infected material because infertility can result from such an infection.

WHAT CAN I DO?

• Whatever the reason for the miscarriage and whatever the treatment your doctor prescribes, the emotional effects can be devastating. In addition to the natural feelings of grief, you will probably feel angry that your body has let you down.

• The one emotion you must try to combat is guilt. It is not your fault and, although you may feel like hiding yourself away and perhaps punishing yourself, this is not the way to get back to normal. Do not isolate yourself and try to be positive about what you can do in the future.

• Anxiety is one of the emotional factors that can result in a failure to conceive. Your doctor should give you an honest answer as soon as possible about whether you can successfully carry a baby to full term without medical treatment. If he says it's possible, keep trying, but try not to become obsessive. If you have a problem that can be treated, don't waste time – seek treatment.

• A miscarriage is a true bereavement and is very difficult to cope with. Counseling might help and is available. If you think you'd benefit from this, ask your doctor to put you in touch with a counselor.

• You can usually resume sexual intercourse within about three weeks, when the bleeding has stopped and the cervix has

TYPES OF MISCARRIAGE

There are several types of first trimester miscarriage (spontaneous abortion):

• *Threatened miscarriage,* where there is spotting of blood, sometimes when the menstrual period would have been due, but the cervix is closed. This does not invariably lead to the loss of the fetus.

• *Inevitable miscarriage,* which is accompanied by more severe vaginal bleeding and pain because the uterus is contracting. Virtually nothing can prevent the expulsion of the fetus. Inevitable miscarriages are either complete (when both the fetus and placenta are expelled) or incomplete (when the fetus is expelled but parts of the placenta remain).

• *Missed abortion,* in which the fetus dies in the uterus but remains there.

• *Recurrent or habitual miscarriage,* in which a woman has three or more miscarriages that have occurred at the same time and for the same reason in each pregnancy.

• *Induced abortion,* in which the pregnancy is terminated by medical means (see p. 85).

closed. You will probably be advised to wait for at least two complete menstrual periods before trying to conceive again.

SEE ALSO:
D&C/ERPC, *page 82*
Fibroids, *page 41*
Hysterosalpingogram, *page 76*
Laparoscopy, *page 77*
Syphilis, *page 56*
Termination of Pregnancy, *page 85*
Ultrasound Scan, *page 75*

ECTOPIC PREGNANCY

When a pregnancy develops in an organ other than the uterus, it is known as an ectopic pregnancy. The most common site is in one of the fallopian tubes, but the fertilized embryo can very occasionally implant on other organs within the pelvis. The egg is fertilized in the fallopian tube, and if the tube is damaged in any way, the egg may become stuck there. Ectopic pregnancies occur in about one out of every hundred pregnancies and are more common in first pregnancies, if you have an IUD, are taking the progesterone-only contraceptive pill, and with postcoital contraception.

SYMPTOMS
- *Missed period, nausea, and fatigue*
- *Colicky type of abdominal pain*
- *Unexpected vaginal bleeding, which could be mistaken for an early miscarriage*
- *Pallor, sweating, and faintness if you have internal bleeding*
- *Sharp shoulder pain*
- *Shock; hot and cold flushes and dizziness*

IS IT SERIOUS?

An ectopic pregnancy is always very serious because the fetus inevitably outgrows the fallopian tube and bursts through it, leading to hemorrhage, shock, pelvic infection, peritonitis, and, if untreated, collapse and death.

SHOULD I SEE THE DOCTOR?

If there is any chance you could be pregnant and you are suffering pain in either the right or left side of your lower abdomen, consult your doctor immediately. Women with a history of **pelvic inflammatory disease** (PID) are particularly at risk. Home pregnancy tests are not reliable in tubal pregnancies, so don't hesitate even if you had a negative result on the test.

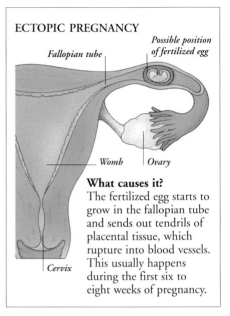

ECTOPIC PREGNANCY

Fallopian tube

Possible position of fertilized egg

Womb | *Ovary*

Cervix

What causes it?
The fertilized egg starts to grow in the fallopian tube and sends out tendrils of placental tissue, which rupture into blood vessels. This usually happens during the first six to eight weeks of pregnancy.

WHAT MIGHT THE DOCTOR DO?

- It is possible your doctor will be able to feel the pregnancy by examining your abdomen externally. **Ultrasound scanning** is also used as a diagnostic procedure.
- If a tubal pregnancy is detected, you will need surgery. A specialist will probably perform a **laparoscopy** prior to removal of the pregnancy. If the ectopic pregnancy has burst, the fallopian tube, possibly even your ovary, will be removed.

ARE THERE ANY COMPLICATIONS?

Even if the surgeon can save the fallopian tube, it may heal with scar tissue, impeding the passage of the ovum on that side.

SEE ALSO:
Contraception, *page 14*
Laparoscopy, *page 77*
Pelvic Inflammatory Disease, *page 46*
Ultrasound Scan, *page 75*

8

INVESTIGATIONS AND OPERATIONS

From time to time, various investigations and operations
will be recommended to us, and it is important in making
a choice between one form of treatment and another that
we understand precisely what is being offered so that we
can decide, with our doctors, which is more appropriate
for us. Here, the common tests of adult female life and the
reasons for them, such as cervical smear and ultrasound, are
explained, and surgical operations such as hysterectomy
are described and their consequences discussed.

PELVIC EXAMINATION

A pelvic examination is a routine diagnostic check on the health of your pelvic organs and should be done regularly after the age of 35. The first part is an external manual examination of the abdomen, followed by an internal examination, first manual and then by speculum. Although it is uncomfortable, a pelvic examination is not painful.

WHY IS IT DONE?

Pelvic examinations are done as a matter of routine in well-woman clinics and as an investigation for symptoms such as irregular bleeding, pelvic pain, and bladder problems. Other reasons include:
• As a general check before you are prescribed any form of contraception: the contraceptive pill, fitting of an IUD, diaphragm, or cervical cap; if a **cervical smear** test is being done; if you have had any bleeding after intercourse.

• To check on any unusual or smelly vaginal discharge so that a sample can be taken for laboratory investigation.
• If you suffer from irregular or unusually heavy menstrual bleeding, any bleeding between menstrual periods, or if you have any pain during intercourse (dyspareunia).
• If you suspect that you might have contracted a venereal disease, with any symptoms of pain when passing urine, or sores on the genital area.
• If your mother took the drug DES during her pregnancy.

HOW IS IT DONE?

• An internal examination is done while you lie on your back or on your side. Your doctor will do a preliminary manual examination by placing one or two fingers inside the vagina and the other hand on top of the abdomen (see the illustration, left). In this way, the doctor can feel a cyst, for example, between her two hands and get some idea of size, shape, and texture.
• The speculum examination is an integral part of an internal pelvic examination. The speculum is a plastic or metal instrument shaped somewhat like a duck's bill, which is inserted into the vagina in order to separate the walls of the vagina so that the cervix can be examined.
• A warm, lubricated speculum is inserted with the blades closed. Once inside your vagina, the blades are gently opened so that the cervix and the walls of the vagina can be checked visually.

PELVIC EXAMINATION

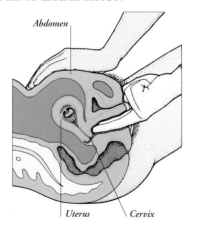

Abdomen

Uterus   Cervix

Manual examination
The size, shape, and any abnormalities of the uterus and other organs, are checked by placing the index and middle fingers inside the vagina and pressing down with the other hand on the abdomen.

SEE ALSO:
Cervical Smear, *page 71*
Contraception, *page 14*
Fertility Problems, *page 59*
Genital Problems, *page 21*
Menstrual Problems, *page 33*
Painful Intercourse, *page 48*
Prolapse, *page 30*
Sexually Transmitted Diseases, *page 51*

CERVICAL SMEAR

Also known as the Pap smear after Dr. Papanicolaou who invented it, this procedure takes place during a routine **pelvic examination**. It is used mainly to detect precancerous and cancerous cells on the cervix.

WHY IS IT DONE?

Cervical smears should be performed on all women once they begin having intercourse and then every year up to the age of 60 – more frequently for women taking the contraceptive pill and those whose mothers were prescribed the drug DES during their pregnancies. The test is also important for those infected with **genital warts**, as this carries a higher risk of cancer. The test also detects urogenital viral infections and sexually transmitted diseases.

HOW IS IT DONE?

• A warmed speculum is passed into the vagina to separate the walls so the doctor can see the condition of your cervix.
• A wooden spatula is wiped across the cervix, and the smear is transferred to a glass slide and sent to a laboratory for analysis.
• The results should be available within six weeks. You should not be menstruating or have had sexual intercourse within 24 hours before your test because blood and semen make the results unreliable.

TEST RESULTS

The results of a smear test are classified into several categories. Negative gives you the all-clear, some mild dysplasia indicates that you have some infection and should be screened more regularly, and a positive smear test, although not always indicating cancer, means there is a detectable change in the cells that necessitates further investigation. Results and the action needed are as follows:
• Negative: No follow-up needed; next smear in one year's time.
• The mildest inflammation known as mild dysplasia, or CIN I: another smear test in

PERFORMING A SMEAR TEST

How is it done?
You lie on your back (right). A speculum is inserted into your vagina then opened to provide a clear view of the cervix.

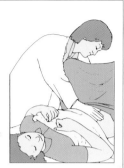

THE PROCEDURE

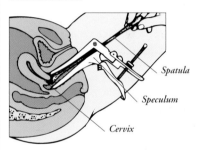

Spatula

Speculum

Cervix

What happens
A spatula is used to scrape cells from the cervix. These are smeared onto a glass slide and sent to a laboratory to be examined. The whole thing takes less than a minute and is not painful.

six months' time.
• More severe inflammation called moderate dysplasia or CIN II: **colposcopy**.
• Severe dysplasia with or without non-invasive cancer, or CIN III: colposcopy with or without **cone biopsy**.

SEE ALSO:
Cervical Cancer, *page 26*
Colposcopy, *page 72*
Cone Biopsy/LETZ, *page 81*
Genital Herpes, *page 52*
Genital Warts, *page 53*
Pelvic Examination, *page 70*

COLPOSCOPY

Colposcopy is the visual examination of the cervix and vagina, usually recommended after a positive **cervical smear**. It is done by using a colposcope, a magnifying instrument that allows the doctor to get a clear, illuminated view of the area.

Colposcopy is a simple, noninvasive procedure and can be used as a treatment as well as a diagnostic tool. It requires no anesthetic and can safely be done in your doctor's office.

WHY IS IT DONE?

A colposcopy is recommended to investigate further any abnormalities indicated by a positive smear or, occasionally, by a **pelvic examination**. The colposcope has a series of powerful lenses that pinpoint much more precisely where any abnormal cells occur, and enables the doctor to obtain a biopsy sample for further investigation.

HOW IS IT DONE?

• The doctor will ask you to remove your lower garments and then to lie on your back with your knees raised and apart, and your feet supported in stirrups.
• A speculum is inserted into your vagina as for a smear test, the vaginal mucus is wiped away, and the area is washed with either a saline solution or a dilute acetic acid. These solutions are used because they cause abnormal cells to show up either white or patterned on the colposcope instead of the usual pink color.
• The colposcope is placed at the entrance to the vagina – it never actually enters the vagina itself. The doctor examines the tissue to identify the precise area of abnormal cells. (A smear test only shows that there is some change but does not pinpoint where.) He will then remove the speculum slowly so that he can inspect the vaginal walls too.
• The procedure takes roughly 15 minutes. Sometimes, using special forceps, your doctor will take a biopsy of abnormal tissue

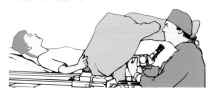

COLPOSCOPY

Telescopic sights
The colposcope is one of the most versatile pieces of equipment in a modern hospital. It is used widely by doctors to monitor pregnancies and pelvic problems, as well as to check on the progress of fertility treatments.

she can see through the lens of the colposcope and this will be sent to a laboratory for further examination.
• If a biopsy is taken, you may have some slight bleeding, but there should be no other side effects.
• If there are abnormal cells inside the cervical canal, a colposcope will not be able to detect them; if this is suspected, a **cone biopsy** will be recommended, to check on cells from inside the canal.
• If a biopsy sample indicates precancerous change only, the affected tissue can be destroyed by laser treatment or by burning away with a hot loop (**LLETZ**).

SEE ALSO:
Cervical Cancer, *page 26*
Cervical Smear, *page 71*
Cone Biopsy/LLETZ, *page 81*
Pelvic Examination, *page 70*

ENDOMETRIAL BIOPSY

Endometrial biopsy involves removing a small amount of tissue from the lining of the uterus (endometrium) in order to examine it for any abnormality. It is a very common procedure, which, while it can be performed under a general anesthetic, is now often done under local anesthetic during an outpatient visit to the hospital.

As a woman gets older, it becomes more difficult in general to obtain an adequate amount of tissue using this technique, and a **hysteroscopy** and **D&C** may be a more appropriate procedure, especially if the abnormal bleeding persists.

WHY IS IT DONE?

The procedure may be carried out to help determine why a woman is suffering from heavy, irregular, or prolonged menstrual periods. If an older woman starts to bleed after menopause, a sample of tissue is also needed to exclude a malignant cause for the bleeding. Occasionally, bleeding after intercourse may lead a doctor to suspect an abnormality in the cells lining the uterus and a biopsy may be performed.

HOW IS IT DONE?

• You will be asked to lie down on a couch in the clinic. A fine plastic "strawlike" instrument is passed into the uterus, via the vagina and cervix, to obtain a piece of tissue that is removed by suction.
• The majority of women tolerate the procedure well; however, some women may find it uncomfortable. Very occasionally the procedure will not be successful, due to a very tight cervix that does not allow the biopsy instrument to pass through it or because the procedure is too uncomfortable for the woman.
• After the biopsy you may find that you have some mild spotting for a day or two. If the investigation was performed with a local anesthetic, you will normally be able to go home immediately afterward.

However, if you have been given a general anesthetic, you will need to stay in the hospital for a few hours to recover.
• The tissue biopsy may take a few weeks to be analyzed by the pathology department. You will normally be seen again in the outpatient department in order to go over the result of the biopsy.
• Depending on what is found, the doctor may decide that no further treatment is required, or she can arrange further investigations, which may include an **ultrasound** examination of the uterus as well as a hysteroscopy and D&C. More extensive surgery, such as a **hysterectomy**, may be necessary if the cells removed from the uterus are found to be malignant.

WHAT CAN I DO?

Discuss with the doctor the exact reasons why it is thought necessary for you to have an endometrial biopsy; don't be afraid to ask questions about anything you are not clear about.

SEE ALSO:
D&C/ERPC, *page 82*
Hysterectomy, *page 79*
Hysteroscopy, *page 74*
Menstrual Problems, *page 33*
Ultrasound Scan, *page 75*
Uterine Cancer, *page 45*

HYSTEROSCOPY

Hysteroscopy involves examining the inside of the uterus with a small telescopic camera that is passed through the cervix. Hysteroscopy can either be performed under a general anesthetic, when it is often combined with a **D&C**, or in the outpatient department. Several types of hysteroscopic procedures have been developed to treat specific problems.

WHY IS IT DONE?

Hysteroscopy is used to examine the inside of the uterus to make sure the lining (endometrium) appears normal, and to check for growths. These may be benign, such as polyps, or malignant. It is an integral part of these investigations to find out the cause of heavy or frequent menstrual periods or bleeding between periods. It is also performed on older women to investigate postmenopausal bleeding.

Hysteroscopy also has a role in removing misplaced or difficult-to-locate IUDs and in the investigation of infertility, to check that the uterus is structurally normal.

HOW IS IT DONE?

• The procedure involves passing the hysteroscope into the cavity of the uterus. If the procedure is being performed in the outpatient clinic you may be given pain medication about 1–2 hours beforehand, and occasionally a local anesthetic will be injected in and around the cervix to help relieve any discomfort.

• In order to obtain a good view of the cavity, it has to be distended using either a harmless gas such as carbon dioxide, or liquid. The doctor will visually inspect the inside of the uterus, making a note of any abnormal areas.

• If it is carried out under a general anesthetic, the procedure is often followed by a D&C.

• Other procedures may be carried out using specially adapted hysteroscopes. The lining of the uterus can be burned away to help treat heavy menstrual periods. This is particularly useful if there is no evidence of malignancy, if drug treatments for heavy periods have been unsuccessful, and to avoid a **hysterectomy**.

• Infertility treatments occasionally use hysteroscopic instruments to divide scar tissue in the uterus and to help correct any congenital structural abnormalities affecting the uterine cavity, including the removal of **fibroids** within the cavity of the uterus.

• For a few days after a hysteroscopy you may notice some spotting of blood. Most women go home the day of the operation. However, some may be required to stay in the hospital for a few days if the hysteroscopy has been combined with an operative procedure.

• In experienced hands, complications of hysteroscopy are uncommon but they can, rarely, include uterine infection and perforation if an additional procedure is being performed, such as endometrial resection.

WHAT CAN I DO?

Make sure that you understand why the procedure is being performed and what will be achieved. Hysteroscopy is usually not performed if you are pregnant and is best avoided if you are suffering from **pelvic inflammatory disease**.

SEE ALSO:

D&C, *page 82*
Fibroids, *page 41*
Hysterectomy, *page 79*
Menstrual Problems, *page 33*
Pelvic Inflammatory Disease, *page 46*

ULTRASOUND SCAN

This is a way of producing a photographic picture by using sound waves. The picture is formed by the echoes of sound waves bouncing off different parts of the body. The echoes differ in their waves according to the density of the organ. Ultrasound scanning can give pictures of soft tissue in great detail. If it is done during pregnancy, it will show fetal heartbeat and movement. An accurate picture of the fetus *in utero* may be printed out that can be used as a noninvasive means of examining the fetus.

Imaging from sound waves
Ultrasound uses sound waves to look inside the body. The waves are converted into electric signals from the recording device and processed by the computer to form a video image on the linked monitor.

WHY IS IT DONE?

Ultrasound is used in many areas of medicine as a diagnostic tool, particularly to detect breast lumps and the cause of abdominal pains, such as gallstones or hiatus hernia. It can also sometimes be used to treat abnormalities. For example, high levels of ultrasound waves can destroy stones in the bladder. In gynecological investigations ultrasound is used:
• To detect endometrial thickness.
• To detect **fibroids**.
• To investigate **uterine cancer**.
• To detect polyps.
• To investigate swollen fallopian tubes.
• To investigate **ovarian cancer**.
• To detect an **ectopic pregnancy**.
Ultrasound scanning is also used widely in fertility treatment and to determine whether a pregnancy is viable or not.

HOW IS IT DONE?

• The procedure is painless and takes about five to ten minutes. It is done when the bladder is full.
• Warm oil is poured over your stomach and a recording device is passed over it by the technician. The device passes back signals that show up on a black and white monitor.
• If you have ultrasound during pregnancy, it is particularly exciting to see your baby in the womb; modern ultrasound monitors can show the baby moving. Ask the technician to point out the head, limbs, and organs to you.

WHAT ARE THE RISKS?

• There appear to be no risks to the unborn child or to the mother, but there is no evidence that it is completely safe either. Therefore, most centers try to use ultrasound sparingly on pregnant women. Scans are only done during pregnancy if doctors and midwives think it advisable.
• If you are extremely worried about something, such as having twins, then your doctor would probably comply with your request for an ultrasound scan. Older women tend to be scanned more frequently.

SEE ALSO:
Ectopic Pregnancy, *page 68*
Fertility Problems, *page 59*
Fibroids, *page 41*
Ovarian Cancer, *page 44*
Uterine Cancer, *page 45*

HYSTEROSALPINGOGRAM

This is an X-ray picture of the womb and fallopian tubes. In the simplest form, the outline of the organs is achieved by pumping up the abdominal cavity with air or carbon dioxide, known as tubal insufflation. This gives a sufficiently clear picture to determine whether the cavity of the uterus is clear and that the fallopian tubes are not blocked. If a more accurate and detailed picture is required, such as precisely where the blockage is, a radio-opaque dye can be injected directly into the uterus and tubes so that their cavities show up on the X ray. If there is no blockage, the dye passes into the cavity and is harmlessly reabsorbed into the body. A blockage of either the uterus or the fallopian tubes can be easily seen because the dye does not flow beyond it.

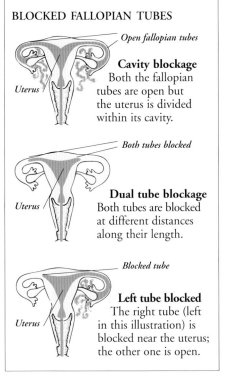

BLOCKED FALLOPIAN TUBES

Open fallopian tubes

Cavity blockage
Both the fallopian tubes are open but the uterus is divided within its cavity.

Uterus

Both tubes blocked

Dual tube blockage
Both tubes are blocked at different distances along their length.

Uterus

Blocked tube

Left tube blocked
The right tube (left in this illustration) is blocked near the uterus; the other one is open.

Uterus

WHY IS IT DONE?

A hysterosalpingogram (HSG) is most commonly used as part of investigations for infertility. It may also be performed after an **ectopic pregnancy** to establish the site and extent of scarring or deformity, or a blockage of the fallopian tubes. The X-ray pictures will show whether there is any distortion in the uterine cavity, such as that caused by a **fibroid** or polyp. It will also show if the fallopian tubes are blocked and pinpoint where the blockage occurs. What it can't do with any accuracy is show the state of the organs, and if there is any doubt remaining after the hysterosalpingogram, the doctor will probably arrange for you to undergo a **laparoscopy** so that the organs can be viewed directly. Laparoscopy has largely replaced HSG because of this.

HOW IS IT DONE?

- Usually HSG takes 10 minutes and can be done either under a local anesthetic or with a sedative but without an anesthetic. It is performed on an outpatient basis, which allows you to go home on the same day.

- Firstly, the cervix is exposed by the insertion of a speculum into the vagina. A hollow metal tube is passed through the cervix, and a radiopaque dye injected into the uterus and X rays taken.

WHAT ARE THE RISKS?

This is not a difficult procedure although, as the dye is injected into the uterus, you may experience some cramping sensations. A hysterosalpingogram is painful, so take pain medication beforehand.

SEE ALSO:
Ectopic Pregnancy, *page 68*
Fertility Problems, *page 59*
Fibroids, *page 41*
Laparoscopy, *page 77*

LAPAROSCOPY

Certain conditions can be diagnosed accurately only if the organs are directly seen. Laparoscopy is a procedure that enables a doctor to see both the inside of the abdominal cavity and organs such as the gallbladder, liver, and uterus through an instrument called a laparoscope.

The most common use of laparoscopy is in gynecology. The procedure is used to view the pelvis and pelvic organs. The long metal tube with a lens and a light at one end and a telescope at the other allows the abdominal cavity to be seen through the telescopic eyepiece.

WHY IS IT DONE?

The advantages of laparoscopy are that the patient suffers less than with other more invasive procedures, and that the surgeon obtains a better view of the internal organs. Laparoscopy is most commonly used for the following:

- Tubal surgery, including **sterilization**.
- Infertility investigations.
- **Ovarian cysts**.
- **Fibroids**.
- **Ectopic pregnancy**.
- Laparoscopic **hysterectomy**.
- Bladder operations for stress incontinence.

HOW IS IT DONE?

- If laparoscopy is for a minor operation such as tubal ligation, you may be offered an epidural anesthetic, but generally it is done under a general anesthetic.
- A tiny cut is made in the abdomen, usually just below the navel so that no scar is visible afterward. A needle is inserted into the abdomen and carbon dioxide gas is pumped into the abdominal cavity so that organs can be visualized.
- The laparoscope is passed in and the doctor can angle it to get a clear view. If other instruments are being used, these are inserted through a second incision above the pubic line.

- The procedure usually takes about 30–40 minutes and you will have one or two stitches in the skin.
- After about two hours, depending on the reason for the laparoscopy, you should be allowed to go home.
- You may have a little discomfort from any gas that remains in your pelvic cavity, and the incision site may be sore. However, laparoscopy is very safe and you should have few problems.

SEE ALSO:

Ectopic Pregnancy, *page 68*
Fertility Problems, *page 59*
Fibroids, *page 41*
Ovarian Cysts, *page 42*
Pelvic Inflammatory Disease, *page 46*
Sterilization, *page 83*

MYOMECTOMY

Myomectomy is the name given to the operation to remove **fibroids**, which are benign growths of muscular tissue in the wall of the uterus. Fibroids, which may be single or multiple, can grow to a large size and may be in the wall of the uterus or within its cavity.

WHY IS IT DONE?

Myomectomy allows the removal of fibroids without the necessity for a **hysterectomy**, so it is most generally reserved for those women who have not yet completed their families. Occasionally, however, if you have large multiple fibroids, or if there is a suspicion of malignancy, your doctor may recommend a hysterectomy rather than a myomectomy even if you have not completed your family.

HOW IS IT DONE?

• Myomectomy is performed under a general anesthetic. The doctor may ask for your agreement in advance for proceeding to a hysterectomy if the myomectomy is too technically difficult.

• Prior to surgery you will probably have an **ultrasound** examination of your uterus to help determine the size and number of fibroids. Some doctors may treat you with special medicines over a period of several months to help shrink the fibroids prior to surgery, especially if they are very bulky. This often helps the surgeon make the smallest possible incision and can minimize blood loss during the operation.

• The operation involves making an incision in the abdomen. This incision is either along the "bikini line" – a Pfannenstiel incision – or occasionally, because of the size of the fibroids, it may be lengthwise (a midline incision), along the center of the abdomen.

• The operation involves making small cuts along the surface of the uterus and then removing each fibroid individually. The operation may take quite a long time to complete, especially if multiple fibroids are found or if they are in particularly difficult-to-reach positions.

• Postoperative management involves an intravenous drip to provide fluid and nutrients, a catheter to help drain away urine, and an abdominal drain to help get rid of any blood that may leak from the uterus. After the operation, you will be required to stay in the hospital for seven to ten days. You will normally be seen in the outpatient department about six weeks after the operation.

ARE THERE ANY SIDE EFFECTS?

• Myomectomy can be a technically difficult operation. Blood loss can be significant, which may mean that a blood transfusion will have to be given. In addition, it does not remove small "seedling" fibroids, which over the years could grow to cause troublesome symptoms again.

• Women who are experiencing difficulties in conceiving because of fibroids must remember that removing fibroids does not necessarily guarantee that a successful pregnancy will be possible.

WHAT CAN I DO?

• You must make sure that you discuss the possibility of a hysterectomy fully with your doctor before surgery is attempted, and come to a mutual understanding.

• Be prepared for a long postoperative recovery period. You will have had a long operation and possibly blood loss, and your body will need time to recover.

SEE ALSO:
Fibroids, *page 41*
Hysterectomy, *page 79*
Menstrual Problems, *page 33*
Ultrasound Scan, *page 75*

HYSTERECTOMY

A hysterectomy is the surgical removal of the uterus. In the United States, 25 percent of all women over 50 have had subtotal or radical hysterectomies (see below). The operation is often performed for no good or compelling reason, such as the removal of small **fibroids**. Some doctors even advocate it once childbearing is over to forestall the risk of uterine or ovarian cancer, but this is totally unjustified. The decision to have a hysterectomy should never be taken lightly and, especially in young women, the instant menopause that results must be treated with HRT.

In Britain, until recently there has been a reluctance by doctors to remove the uterus unless the symptoms really warranted it, and not without full discussion and perhaps a second opinion.

WHY IS IT DONE?

The operation is undertaken for the following reasons:
• To remove cancer in the pelvic organs.
• To treat any severe and uncontrollable pelvic infection.
• To stop severe hemorrhage.
• In certain conditions affecting the intestines and bladder that threaten a woman's life, when it is impossible to deal with the primary problem without removal of the uterus.
• Multiple fibroids that are causing bleeding and pain.
• The operation is sometimes done to treat **prolapse**; as a method of **sterilization**; to treat severe **endometriosis**; because of injury to the pelvic muscles at childbirth, severe enough to interfere with bowel and bladder function; and for uncontrollable uterine bleeding.

WHAT SHOULD I DO?

• Question your doctor very carefully about the reasons for your hysterectomy and be satisfied in your mind that it is absolutely necessary. Explore all the possible alternatives, and involve your partner and family fully.
• Check to see whether your ovaries need to be removed as well as your uterus, and find out about hormone replacement treatments available for premature menopause if your surgeon insists they should be removed. It is no longer medically accepted that ovaries should be removed in case cancer should develop, so don't be persuaded by this argument.

TYPES OF HYSTERECTOMY

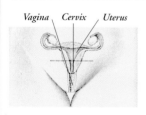

Vagina *Cervix* *Uterus*

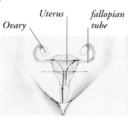

Uterus *fallopian tube*
Ovary

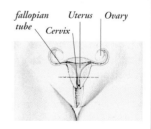

fallopian tube *Uterus* *Ovary*
Cervix

Radical hysterectomy
The uterus, cervix, surrounding tissue, lymph glands, part of the vagina, fallopian tubes, and ovaries are all removed.

Subtotal hysterectomy
Only the uterus is removed in a subtotal hysterectomy.

Total hysterectomy
The uterus and cervix are removed in a total hysterectomy. The ovaries and fallopian tubes are left behind.

HYSTERECTOMY: CONTINUED

HOW IS IT DONE?

• For the abdominal route, an incision is made under general anesthetic in the lower abdomen, and then the uterus, and possibly the ovaries and fallopian tubes, too, are removed.

• After the operation you will have an intravenous drip for fluids or blood, and perhaps a catheter to drain urine. There will be some discharge from the vagina for a day or two after the operation.

• If your ovaries were removed, hormone replacement treatment will be planned. You will be encouraged to get out of bed after a couple of days.

• Alternatively, you may have a vaginal hysterectomy, in which the abdominal cavity isn't opened but the uterus is removed through the vagina. A woman's recovery is quicker this way and the complications are either minimized or avoided altogether. This is the ideal operation to correct uncomplicated uterine prolapse. Vaginal hysterectomy is only performed if the uterus is not too bulky and if the supporting structures are not too tight.

• An incision is made in the uterus and high in the roof of the vagina, and, if necessary, the ovaries are removed from below.

• The normal hospital stay is five days, and you will be seen in the outpatient department six weeks later. Provided that there are no problems, intercourse can be resumed after this visit.

• A combination approach called LAVH (laparoscopic assisted vaginal hysterectomy) has now become more common. The technique involves using a laparoscope inserted into the abdominal cavity to help perform the operation vaginally.

WHAT CAN I DO?

• When you go home after the operation, maintain a moderate level of activity, but stop the minute you feel pain.

• Gradually build up your strength. Gentle activities can be started by the fourth week after the operation; moderate activity like light shopping or housework can be undertaken by the fifth week. By the sixth week you should feel nearly back to normal, although you may still feel fatigued.

• By the eighth week you can resume sexual intercourse, since the top of the vagina will have healed. There is no reason why sex should be any different for you; many women report increased satisfaction.

ARE THERE PSYCHOLOGICAL CHANGES?

• Nearly half of women who have hysterectomies are satisfied with the operation. The vagina will be the same size as it was before, unless the operation was a radical hysterectomy (see p. 79).

• Dissatisfaction is related to whether the operation was done for a very good reason and after full consideration by the woman of the options available.

• Women who want more children find it difficult, as do those whose ovaries are removed premenopausally.

• The majority of women who suffer depression after hysterectomy are those for whom the operation was undertaken for a condition that was not life-threatening. It seems easier to bear if you know that the operation saved your life.

SEE ALSO:
Cervical Cancer, *page 26*
Endometriosis, *page 40*
Fibroids, *page 41*
Laparoscopy, *page 77*
Ovarian Cancer, *page 44*
Pelvic Inflammatory Disease, *page 46*
Prolapse, *page 30*
Sterilization, *page 83*
Uterine Cancer, *page 45*

CONE BIOPSY/LLETZ

A cone biopsy, or conization, is one of the methods used to remove suspect tissue from the cervix for investigation or treatment. It is also known as LLETZ (large loop excision of the transformation zones). **Colposcopy** is the less invasive method of diagnosis and, where available, is preferable for investigating and diagnosing any changes to cervical tissue.

WHY IS IT DONE?

A cone biopsy is performed if one or more **cervical smear** tests indicate dysplasia or the presence of cancerous cells in the cervix. Dysplasia (cell abnormality) occurs if the skin on the outside of the cervix changes. This is symptomless and presents no risk to your health, although in some cases cancer develops after a long period of time. It is detected as the result of a routine cervical smear test when some change in the cells is noted. Cone biopsy is performed if a colposcopy has failed to pinpoint the location of the diseased cells. This is most likely to be the case for women over 35, since less of their cervical tissue can be seen on inspection due to retraction caused by age, or when the full extent of suspicious cells cannot be determined accurately.

HOW IS IT DONE?

A cone biopsy is usually performed under a general anesthetic. The entire area of affected tissue, usually cone-shaped, hence its name, is removed with a scalpel or laser beam. Often a **D&C** will be performed at the same time to check the lining of the uterus for any spread of cancer. The area will be sutured by using diathermy (intense heat) or freezing to reduce bleeding, although it can also be stitched. The tissue is then sliced and examined microscopically to confirm the diagnosis. Although used as a diagnostic tool for **cervical cancer**, a cone biopsy can result in successful treatment if the entire cancerous area is removed. If this is not so, further surgery or radiation therapy will be required.

WHAT HAPPENS AFTERWARD?

You will be able to remain in the hospital for two or three days. There will probably be some bleeding and this may be stopped by packing your vagina with gauze. If the bleeding recurs, consult your doctor. You will still require regular smear tests.

ARE THERE ANY RISKS?

There is some risk to the cervix with this procedure; the cervical canal may narrow, bringing about some reduction in fertility. Carbon dioxide laser has recently been introduced as another means of removing tissue for analysis. The risk of bleeding and other complications is reduced by using this method and it can also be performed on an outpatient basis.

CONE BIOPSY

Affected area of the cervix

Cone of cervix tissue

Cervical biopsy
After the area of the cervix containing the abnormal cells is removed (above right), the wound is closed by stitching, diathermy (heat), or cryosurgery (freezing).

SEE ALSO:
Cervical Cancer, *page 26*
Cervical Smear, *page 71*
Colposcopy, *page 72*
D&C/ERPC, *page 82*

D&C/ERPC

D&C (dilatation and curettage) is a gynecological procedure in which the lining of the uterus (endometrium) is scraped away. A form of D&C (in effect a curettage without dilatation) is carried out after an incomplete abortion, when it is called an ERPC (evacuation of the retained products of conception). ERPC is carried out after a **hysteroscopy** has identified what remains in the uterus. A D&C is usually performed under a brief general anesthetic, on a hospital outpatient basis.

WHY IS IT DONE?

These days, a D&C is usually done to remove the lining of the womb in order to find out the cause of heavy menstrual bleeding (**menorrhagia**), or for other uterine problems such as polyps or misplaced intrauterine coils (IUDs).

In scraping away the lining, D&C can treat the problems it finds at the same time. It was traditionally used as a means of terminating an early pregnancy, although it is very rarely employed for this purpose these days.

HOW IS IT DONE?

• First, a speculum is inserted into the vagina to separate the vaginal walls so that the cervix can be seen. A series of rods are then inserted to dilate the cervix.
• If the procedure is being performed to check for polyps, the cervix is dilated and a polyps forceps explores the uterine cavity, grasping and removing any polyps that are found. Finally a spoon-shaped instrument, the curette, is inserted into the womb to scrape away the lining.
• The scrapings from the curette are examined for abnormalities under a microscope in a laboratory.
• After the D&C you will need to rest and recover for several hours before going home. You should take it easy for a day or so afterward, but you shouldn't experience any problems. You can resume sexual relations within a week or so, or whenever you feel comfortable. Your menstrual cycle will recommence within about six weeks.
• To perform an ERPC after an incomplete abortion, the procedure varies a little. There is usually no need to dilate the cervix (it will remain open if any conception material remains), so a sponge forceps is used with a curette to gently clean out the placenta and any fetal material.

DILATATION AND CURETTAGE

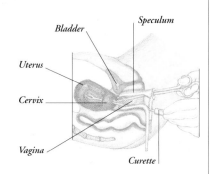

Bladder
Speculum
Uterus
Cervix
Vagina
Curette

A simple procedure
For dilatation, a speculum holds the vaginal walls apart while rods are inserted into the cervix to dilate it. For curettage, a curette is inserted into the womb and the walls are carefully scraped with it.

SEE ALSO:
Endometriosis, *page 40*
Fibroids, *page 41*
Hysteroscopy, *page 74*
Menorrhagia, *page 38*
Menstrual Problems, *page 33*
Miscarriage, *page 66*
Termination of Pregnancy, *page 85*

STERILIZATION

This is a supposedly permanent surgical means of birth control that makes it impossible for an egg to be fertilized and conception to take place.

The simplest sterilization is carried out on men. It involves tying the tubes (*vas deferens*) that connect the testicles to the penis. Ejaculate is still emitted during orgasm, but it contains no sperm and therefore is not capable of fertilizing an ovum. This operation is called a vasectomy and is performed under a local anesthetic in about 20 minutes. It does not affect virility and sexual performance, nor does it increase susceptibility to illness.

In women, the usual method is tubal ligation, which closes off the fallopian tubes. This creates an obstruction that keeps the ovum from moving through to the uterus or sperm from reaching the ovum, thereby preventing conception from taking place.

WHY IS IT DONE?

Sterilization is usually only performed on men or women who have already had children and do not want to have more. Since it is a permanent operation that is very difficult to reverse, doctors are generally unwilling to sterilize childless women or women under 30.

For some women the decision is a difficult one. While they may be freed from the fear of having an unwanted pregnancy, they need to come to terms with their feelings about taking this irrevocable step. They may also have to deal with their partner's refusal to have a vasectomy, which is a far less invasive procedure.

HOW IS IT DONE?

• There are several different methods of female sterilization, using either the abdominal or vaginal approach. All are carried out under general anesthetic or occasionally an epidural.

• Carbon dioxide gas may be introduced into the abdomen to inflate it so that the internal organs can be more clearly seen. While all the procedures involve tying or closing the tubes in some way, a small portion of the tube itself is almost invariably removed.

• Some other forms of surgery, such as **hysterectomy**, result in sterilization, but these operations should never be used solely for this purpose.

• The tubes are either tied or cut, clamped with rings or clips, plugged, or frozen. This can be carried out by means of laparotomy, culdoscopy, or **laparoscopy**.

STERILIZATION

Male sterilization
In vasectomy, the *vas deferens* (the tube that carries sperm from the testes) is cut in two, and the ends bent back and closed to prevent the tube from reforming.

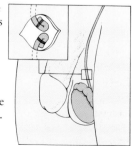

Female sterilization

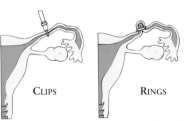

CLIPS   RINGS

Two common ways to carry out female sterilizations are to clip the fallopian tubes or to close them with a tight elastic ring.

STERILIZATION: CONTINUED

Mini-laparotomy

First, a slim surgical tool is inserted into the vagina to manipulate the top of the uterus close to the abdominal wall. The surgeon then makes a small incision – about 1in (2.5cm) – into the abdomen, near the uterus, lifts out each fallopian tube in turn, and clips and ties it.

Laparoscopy

This is the most commonly used technique to perform tubal ligation. A laparoscope, which contains a fiber-optic filament, is inserted into the abdomen, often through a tiny incision in the navel and, under direct vision, the fallopian tubes are clamped. The hospital stay should only be one day, but laparoscopy can be done on an outpatient basis at some clinics.

Culdoscopy

In this procedure, an incision is made in the vagina just below the cervix. A clamp on the cervix is used to position the uterus so that the tubes can be seen. The tubes are then brought down one at a time, cut, tied, clipped, or blocked.

WHAT ARE THE AFTEREFFECTS?

• After the sterilization, you won't notice any change in your normal menstrual pattern, and you will have a normal menopause when it occurs because your ovaries have not been affected by the procedure. The ovum produced every month will be absorbed into the body rather than being expelled, as it would have been normally when fertilization did not occur.

• Some women have a routine **D&C** when they are sterilized; this is a check of the uterus for any growths or problems. Usually there is bleeding from the vagina for a day or two and some local discomfort at the site of any incision. You may also notice pain in your shoulder, caused by irritation from the carbon dioxide gas.

• You may also have a reaction to the general anesthetic. If you've had a reaction to a general anesthetic during previous surgery, suggest to your doctor that an epidural might be used.

• If you had a vaginal sterilization, you will not be able to have intercourse for a couple of weeks because of the danger of infection, but you'll have no external scar.

WHAT ARE THE RISKS?

There are few serious risks or complications with any of the methods of sterilization described here, except those normally expected of any surgical procedure. Tubal ligation by the vaginal route has a slightly increased risk of infection.

IS IT EFFECTIVE?

• Sterilization has a higher efficiency rate than any other means of contraception and it is permanent. After the operation no other form of birth control is necessary.

• The operation is considered irreversible, although microsurgery, in a few cases, has succeeded in sewing the tubes back together again. There will be no effect on your libido or sex life.

• Men often feel their potency has been interfered with after vasectomy; but this is only in the mind and has no basis in reality.

SEE ALSO:
Contraception, *page 14*
D&C/ERPC, *page 82*
Hysterectomy, *page 79*
Laparoscopy, *page 77*

TERMINATION OF PREGNANCY

With changes in attitudes to termination of pregnancy, this is now legally performed in the United States before the 24th week of pregnancy, for both medical and psychological reasons. In some countries, abortion is illegal, and even in those countries where it is allowed, the terms under which it is performed and the time of gestation differ considerably depending on where you live.

Unfortunately there are still many myths about terminating a pregnancy, which may be dangerous. If you are considering terminating a pregnancy, remember that:

• There is nothing you can take by mouth that will safely and efficiently result in a termination of pregnancy.
• Hot baths, bottles of gin, and jumping from a great height will not cause abortion if the fetus and placenta are healthy.
• Procuring an illegal abortion may result in heavy bleeding. Any heavy bleeding should be treated immediately. There may be some retained placenta or an infection that should be treated as an emergency.

WHAT ARE THE RISKS?

Medically induced abortion, whether legal or illegal, brings the following risks:
• Infection of the uterus.
• Infection of the fallopian tubes.
• Blockage of the fallopian tubes leading to subfertility or infertility.
• An increased likelihood of an **ectopic pregnancy** later.
• The cervix becomes so stretched that it becomes incompetent.
• Perforation of the uterus.
• Retained placenta leading to hemorrhage and risk of death.

WHY IS IT DONE?

Women seek abortions for many different reasons, and these can include: personal or financial reasons; failed contraception; medical tests that have shown the fetus to be abnormal; and rape. With sophisticated prenatal tests, more damaged babies are being discovered in early pregnancy. When the results of the tests are known, the parents of the unborn child are usually offered counseling, which will include discussion about termination.

Medical reasons for abortion would be:
• Continuing the pregnancy involves greater risk to your life than the abortion.
• Continuing the pregnancy involves a greater risk of injury to the physical and mental health of your living children than termination.
• There is a substantial risk that the child will be born seriously deformed or suffering from a life-threatening disorder such as hemophilia or cystic fibrosis.
• Trauma and unnecessary misery would result from the birth of a child conceived through rape.

HOW IS IT DONE?

Try to plan far enough ahead so that the abortion can be performed at the best time, before the 14th week of pregnancy, and preferably before 12 weeks. After 14 weeks, the procedure is not only more difficult but also more dangerous.

At this later stage, termination is induced with prostaglandins that result in an abortion within 12–36 hours. It can be very painful, like labor. Unfortunately, even when an abortion has been approved, waiting lists for the procedure can cause you to wait until you are more than 16 weeks pregnant, and only an induced labor is open to you.

Suction termination (4–8 weeks)
• This is a very early termination and may be carried out with a local anesthetic if it is sufficiently early in the pregnancy. It is certainly the safest and least traumatic form of termination. It takes about five minutes and can be done in a doctor's office, clinic, or outpatient department in the hospital.

TERMINATION OF PREGNANCY: CONTINUED

• A small tube is inserted through the vagina into the uterus. A syringe or pump gently sucks out the uterine lining and fetal material through the tube.

ERPC (After 4 weeks)

• As above, but an ERPC is carried out under general anesthetic or epidural. The procedure takes about 30 minutes and recovery will involve some painful cramps.
• You may be given medicines to help the uterus contract afterward to reduce bleeding and the possibility of infection.

Induced labor termination (16–24 weeks)

• By 16 weeks the walls of the uterus are thinner and can be perforated more easily. The fetus is larger, so an induced labor with its attendant emotional and physical pain is usually necessary.
• A cervagen or mifepristone pill is given to induce labor. You will have painful contractions and should be offered pain medication. You may be given a hormone such as oxytocin to increase contractions. The fetus and placenta are expelled relatively easily. The fetus is recognizable and may live for a few minutes, which is upsetting.
• You may then have an ERPC to check that there is nothing left in your uterus, and medication to suppress lactation will be given to you. You will probably stay in the hospital for about three days but, because of the shortage of hospital beds, you may be in wards with women who have had babies or those who cannot. This is upsetting and you should seek to avoid this if possible.

Hysterotomy (16–24 weeks)

This is rarely performed because it is a major operation requiring a general anesthetic. It is only used for women who cannot have prostaglandin treatment or for whom the other methods have been unsuccessful.

AFTER A TERMINATION

What happens to you after your termination depends very much on you, and on the stage of pregnancy you were at when you underwent the procedure. The following are sensible guidelines to bear in mind in the days immediately after the procedure.

• Get treatment immediately if you have any heavy bleeding, severe abdominal pain, or a smelly vaginal discharge.
• Your menstrual period should probably resume within a month to six weeks of the operation. Don't use tampons for the first menstrual period.
• Abstain from sexual intercourse while you still have spot bleeding after the procedure (this should disappear after a few days); thereafter you can resume whenever you feel comfortable doing so.
• An early abortion should mean that you are back to normal physically within a week. For a later termination (after 16 weeks), allow two to three weeks.
• Even if you don't think you need it, you would be wise to seek some counseling after a termination; suppressed guilt, shame, and regret can be traumatic and damaging – and can potentially affect current and future relationships if they aren't dealt with.
• Have a checkup six weeks after the termination.
• Start using some form of contraception immediately.

It is like a cesarean section when the fetus is removed through an incision in the abdominal wall and uterus.

SEE ALSO:
Ectopic Pregnancy, *page 68*
D&C/ERPC, *page 82*
Miscarriage, *page 66*

USEFUL ADDRESSES

The organizations listed below are among many that provide information on women's health issues. Most included in this list provide information either by phone or via the internet; others will send printed information in answer to queries.

AGING

American Geriatrics Society
770 Lexington Avenue,
New York, NY 10021
Tel: (212) 308-1414
http://www.americangeriatrics. org

Older Women's League
666 11th Street NW,
Washington, DC 20001
Tel: (800) TAKE-OWL/
(202) 783-6686

AIDS AND SEXUALLY TRANSMITTED DISEASES

American Social Health Association
PO Box 13827
Research Triangle Park,
NC 27009
Tel: (800) 342-AIDS (AIDS hotline)/(919) 361-8488 (herpes hotline)
http://www.sunsite.unc.edu/ ASHA

SIECUS (Sex Information and Education Council of the US)
130 West 42nd Street,
New York, NY 10036
Tel: (212) 819-9770

Women Alive
1566 S. Burnside Avenue
Los Angeles, CA 90019
Tel: (213) 965-1564
http://www.thebody.com/wa/ wapage.html

GENERAL HEALTH

American College of Obstetricians and Gynecologists
Resource Center
409 12th Street SW
Washington, DC 20024-2188
Tel: (202) 863-2518

The American Medical Association
515 North State Street
Chicago, IL 60610
Tel: (312) 464-5000
http://www.ama-assn.org

Centers for Disease Control and Prevention
1600 Clifton Road NE
Atlanta, GA 30333
(404) 639-3311
http://www.cdc.gov

Lupus Foundation of America
4 Research Place,
Rockville, MD 20850-3226
Tel: (800) 558-0121/
(301) 670-9292
http://www.lupus.org/lupus

Med Help International
Suite 130, Box 188
6300 North Wickham Road
Melbourne, FL 32940
Tel: (407) 253-9048
http://www.medhelp.org

National Institutes of Health
9000 Rockville Pike
Bethesda, MD 20892
Tel: (301) 496-4000
http://www.nih.gov

National Kidney and Urologic Diseases
Information Clearinghouse
Three Information Way
Bethesda, MD 20892-3580
Tel: (301) 654-4415
http://www.niddk.nih.gov

National Osteoporosis Foundation
1150 17th Street NW
Washington, DC 20036
Tel: (800) 223-9994/
(202) 223-2226
http://www.nof.org

National Women's Health Network
514 10th Street NW,
Washington, DC 20004
Tel: (202) 347-1140

US Food and Drug Administration (FDA)
Office of Consumer Affairs
Inquiry Information Line
Tel: (301) 827-4420
http://www.fda.gov

MENTAL HEALTH

American Counseling Association
5999 Stevenson Avenue
Alexandria, VA 22304
Tel: (800) 347-6647/
(703) 823-9800
http://www.counseling.org

National Mental Health Association
1021 Prince Street
Alexandria, VA 22314-2971
Tel: (800) 969-NMHA/
(703) 684-7722
http://www.nmisp.org

CANCER

American Cancer Society
1599 Clifton Road NE
Atlanta, GA 30329
Tel: (800) ACS-2345/
(404) 320-3333
http://www.cancer.org

Cancer Care, Inc.
1180 Avenue of the Americas
New York, NY 10036
Tel: (800) 813-HOPE/
(212) 221-3300
http://www.cancercareinc.org

HERS (Hysterectomy Educational Resources and Services)
422 Bryn Mawr Avenue
Bala Cynwyd, PA 19004
Tel: (610) 667-7757
http://www.dca.net/~hers/

National Alliance of Breast Cancer Organizations
9 East 37th Street, 10th Floor
New York, NY 10016
Tel: (800) 719-9154/
(212) 889-0606
http://www.nabco.org

National Cancer Institute
31 Center Drive MSC 2580
9000 Rockville Pike
Bethesda, MD 20892-2580
Tel: (800) 4-CANCER/
(301) 496-5583

Strang Cancer Prevention Center
428 East 72nd Street
New York, NY 10021
Tel: (800) 521-9356/
(212) 794-4900

The Susan G. Komen Breast Cancer Foundation
5005 LBJ Freeway,
Dallas, TX 75244
Tel: (800) 462-9273/
(972) 233-0351

The Skin Cancer Foundation
245 Fifth Avenue
New York, NY 10016
Tel: (800) SKIN-490/
(212) 725-5176
e-mail: info@skincancer.org

Y-ME: National Breast Cancer Organization
212 W. Van Buren Street
Chicago, IL 60607-3908
Tel: (800) 221-2141/
(312) 986-8228/
(312) 986-8338
http://www.Y-ME.org

FERTILITY

America's Crisis Pregnancy Helpline
2121 Valley View Lane
Dallas, TX 75234
Tel: (800) 67-BABY6/
(214) 241-BABY
e-mail: acph@dallas.net

Ferre Institute, Inc.
258 Genessee Street,
Utica, NY 13502
Tel: (315) 724-4348
e-mail: ferreinf@aol.com

Maternity Center Association
281 Park Avenue South,
New York, NY 10010
Tel: (212) 777-5000

The National Coalition for Birthing Alternatives
4755 West Avenue, L-13
Quartz Hill, CA 93536
http://www.ptw.com/~troytash

Resolve
1310 Broadway
Somerville, MA 02144-1799
Tel: (617) 623-0744
http://www.resolve.org

CONTRACEPTION

Association for Voluntary Sterilization
125 Park Avenue
New York, NY 10017
Tel: (212) 557-6600

Planned Parenthood Federation of America
810 Seventh Avenue
New York, NY 10017
Tel: (212) 541-7800
http://www.plannedparenthood.org

COMPLEMENTARY MEDICINE

American Academy of Osteopathy
3500 DePauw Boulevard,
Indianapolis, IN 46268
Tel: (317) 879-1881
http://www.aao.medguide.net.com

American Holistic Health Association (A.H.H.A.)
PO Box 17400
Anaheim, CA 92817-7400
Tel: (714) 779-6152
http://www.ahha.org

American Osteopathic Association
142 East Ontario Street
Chicago, IL 60611
Tel: (312) 202-8000
http://www.am-osteo-assn.org

Center for Complementary and Alternative Medicine Research in Women's Health
Columbia University
630 West 168th Street
New York, NY 10032
http://www.cpmcnet.columbia.edu/dept/rosenthal

Office of Alternative Medicine National Institutes of Health
PO Box 8218
Silver Spring, MD 20907
Tel: (888) 644-6226

GLOSSARY

Acupuncture
A system of treatment in which needles are inserted into the skin and either left or manipulated for several minutes. Acupuncturists are not usually medical doctors.

Acute
A term used to describe an illness or pain that comes on suddenly. Acute attacks may be brief but are usually quite severe.

Allergen
Any substance that is normally harmless but provokes an allergic reaction in susceptible individuals. Common allergens include certain foods, animal fur, pollen, or even specks of dust.

Allergy
A reaction to an allergen. Allergies occur as the result of an inappropriate response by the immune system to otherwise harmless substances. Allergic ailments include asthma.

Analgesic
A painkilling medication; aspirin is a common analgesic.

Anesthetic
A medication used to produce a loss of sensation and hence pain in medical and surgical procedures. Anesthetics can be *local*, where the numb sensation is confined to the area of the body being operated upon, or *general*, when it produces

complete unconsciousness. The former is given for relatively minor procedures, while the latter is reserved for more major operations.

Aneurysm
A swelling that occurs if a blood vessel or the heart wall becomes weakened and balloons outward as a result of pressure of the blood within it.

Antibiotic
A medication used to treat bacterial infections. Penicillin is one of the most commonly used antibiotics.

Antibodies
Complex substances produced by special types of white blood cells to neutralize or destroy antigens ("foreign" proteins in the body, such as bacteria; see below). The formation of antibodies against these invading organisms is part of the body's defense against infection.

Antifungal
A medication that is prescribed to treat fungal infections, such as **thrush**.

Antigen
Any substance that can be detected by the body's immune system. Detection usually stimulates production of antibodies.

Antihistamine
A medication that is used to block the effects of *histamines*, chemicals that

are released during the course of an allergic reaction.

Antiseptic
Chemicals that destroy bacteria and other micro-organisms, thereby preventing *sepsis* (infection).

Aspiration
A surgical procedure in which fluid or other matter is sucked from a body cavity by means of an instrument such as a tube or syringe. Aspiration can be used to carry out early **termination of pregnancy**.

Benign
A term used to describe a mild form of a complaint or disease. A benign growth such as a cyst or polyp will neither spread to surrounding tissues nor recur after it has been removed. The opposite, a malignant or cancerous growth, may do both of the above.

Biopsy
A medical procedure during which a small piece of tissue is removed from anywhere in the body for further miscroscopic analysis. Biopsies are usually carried out in order to determine whether or not a growth is malignant or benign. **Cone biopsy** and **endometrial biopsy** are examples.

Blood count
A diagnostic test of a specimen of blood in order to determine the numbers

of the various cells (white, red, and platelets) within a standard volume.

Carcinoma

The most common type of cancer. This malignant growth is composed of abnormally multiplying surface or gland tissue of any organ.

Catheter

A flexible tube used to inject liquid into the body or to drain liquid (urine, for example) from it.

Cauterization

The destruction of tissue (e.g. growths such as warts) by burning away with caustic chemical or a red-hot instrument, or by diathermy.

Chancre

An ulcerated, swollen, painless lump. Can be an early symptom of **syphilis**.

Chemotherapy

The treatment of a disease or cancer by a course of specially selected drugs.

Chronic

A term used to describe a condition that has been present for some time.

Congenital

A term used for a disease or condition present at birth.

Contagious

The term used to describe a disease, such as influenza or measles – that is spread by ordinary social contact.

Cyst

An abnormal growth filled with fluid or solid material that can be located in any organ or tissue, such as the ovaries or cervix.

Diathermy

A procedure that uses a high-frequency hot electric current to destroy or cauterize body tissues. The electric current can burn away the tissue it touches without causing bleeding.

Diuretic

Any substance that increases urine production, thus reducing the fluid content of the body.

Drip

The nonmedical term for an intravenous infusion. A fluid is injected into the body by letting it flow down into a vein from an elevated, sterile container. The rate of flow is measured by counting the rate of dripping.

Embryo

The term used to describe an unborn child up to eight weeks after conception. Thereafter, it is known as a fetus for the remainder of the pregnancy.

Endoscope

An instrument that enables a doctor to look into a body cavity. The basic instrument is a tube equipped with a lighting and lens system, to which various attachments, such as a camera or forceps, can be fixed. Different types

of endoscopes designed for use in specific parts of the body have special names – for example, a laparoscope is used to examine the abdominal cavity.

Hormone

A chemical released directly into the blood stream by a gland or tissue. The body produces many different types of hormone, each of which has a specific range of functions – for instance, estrogen and progesterone control the menstrual cycle.

Immune system

A collection of cells and proteins that recognizes potentially harmful invading organisms, such as bacteria and viruses, and protects the body against them.

Infectious

A term used to describe an illness that is spread by disease-carrying organisms, such as bacteria and viruses. In practice, most sufferers catch infectious diseases through sexual contact, contaminated food, or water or airborne droplets. Diseases such as **AIDS** and meningitis are infectious.

Keratin

A hard or horny substance present in skin, hair, nails, and teeth.

Laser beam

An intensified, controlled beam of light powerful enough to cut or fuse body tissues. Laser beams can be precisely focused for use in delicate operations such as those carried out in eye surgery, and in treatment of cervical abnormalities.

Lymph

A diluted form of plasma that seeps from blood vessels into tissues and delivers nutrients to local cells. Lymph collects in thin-walled vessels and eventually drains back into the circulation, carrying with it waste products from the cells.

Lymph gland

A bean-shaped organ at the junction of several lymph vessels. Each of the many lymph glands in the human body contains thousands of white blood cells for combating invading organisms in the lymph as it passes through the gland.

Mammography

An X-ray procedure used to detect any breast abnormalities in women. All women are advised to have a mammogram once every three years to protect them from breast cancer.

Menarche

The onset of menstruation. Menarche usually occurs between the ages of about 12 and 15.

Oophorectomy

The removal of one or both ovaries. This operation is now usually performed as part of a **hysterectomy**.

Pessary

A device placed in the vagina. Pessaries are used to treat genital complaints such as **thrush** and can also be used to help induce a **termination of pregnancy**.

Polyp

A swelling that grows, usually on a short stalk, from the wall of a cavity, such as the uterus, or from the skin.

Pus

A thick fluid, usually yellow or greenish, composed of dead white blood cells, decomposed tissue, and bacteria. A collection of pus within solid tissue is called an abscess.

Radiation therapy

A course of treatment that uses either radioactivity or X rays. Radiation therapy is used to destroy malignant, cancerous growths and to slow down or stop the spread of abnormal cells.

Sarcoma

A malignant tumor composed of diseased connective tissue. Sarcomas originate in bones, cartilage, fibrous, or muscular tissues. All types are rare and tend to be difficult to treat.

Secondary

A term applied to a condition, often a malignant growth, that develops as a result of spreading (metastasis) from an earlier (primary) tumor.

Tissue

A collection of cells specialized to perform a specific task in the body, for example connective tissue, where the cells are programed to hold the body together.

Ulcer

An open sore on any external or internal surface of the body. The tissues of an ulcerous area rot away, and pus is likely to ooze from the sore.

Venereal

A term usually applied to disease caused by, or resulting from, some form of sexual contact.

Wart

A common, contagious growth on the skin or mucous membranes. Warts affect only the topmost layer of skin. **Genital warts** are soft warts that grow in and around the entrance of the vagina and anus and on the penis. They are transmitted by sexual contact.

X rays

Rays with a short wavelength that enables them to pass through body tissues. An X-ray photograph resembles the negative of an ordinary photograph, with dense tissues such as bones showing up as white shapes. X rays with very short wavelengths, which can penetrate tissues deeply enough to destroy them, are used in radiation therapy.

INDEX

A

abdominal cramps *see*
dysmenorrhea, 37;
miscarriage, 66; uterine
cancer, 45
abdominal pain *see* chlamydia,
54; cystitis 28;
endometriosis, 40; fibroids,
41; ovarian cancer, 44;
ovarian cysts, 42; PID, 46
abortion, 85–86
induced, 67
missed, 66, 67
septic, 67
spontaneous, 66
acupuncture, 89
acute conditions, 90
adhesiolysis, 40
AIDS, 57–58
allergens, 89
allergies, 89
amenorrhea, 35
anal rash, 24
anemia, 38
anesthetic, 89
anorexia nervosa, 35
anterior repair, 30
antibiotics, 89
antibodies, 89
antihistamines, 89
aromatherapy, 20
aspirin, as prostaglandin
inhibitor, 34, 37
assisted conception,
63–65

B

backache *see* dysmenorrhea,
37; fibroids, 41;
miscarriage, 66; PID, 46;
prolapse, 30, 31
barrier devices, 15–16
basal body temperature
(BBT) charts, 62, 64
Billings method, 14
biopsies, 89
cone, 26, 71, 81
endometrial, 73

birth, giving, 9
bladder:
inability to control, 32
inflammation of, 28
bladder prolapse, 30
bleeding, abnormal, 36
blood count, 89
body, female, 8–9
bones, fragile, 9
bowel movements,
uncomfortable, 30
breast cancer, 18
breast-feeding and
contraception, 14–15
breasts, enlargement of, 10
breathlessness, 44

C

cancer:
AIDS-related, 57
breast, 18
cervical, 26–27, 52
endometrial, 45
ovarian,18, 44
uterine, 18, 41, 45
Candida albicans, 24
carcinoma, 90
caps, cervical, 15, 16
catheters, 28, 90
cauterization, 90
cervical cancer, 26–27, 52
cervical caps, 15, 16
cervical erosion, 23, 36
cervical polyps, 23
cervical smear screening, 26,
27, 52, 71
cervix, 10
incompetent, 66
removal of, 27
chancre, 90
chemotherapy, 44, 90
chlamydia, 46, 54
CIN, 26–27
climacteric, 8, 18
coitus interruptus, 9
colporrhaphy, 30
colposcopy, 26, 71, 72, 81
combined contraceptive pill,
14, 16, 17

complementary therapies, 20
conception, 12–13
assisted, 63–65
condoms, 11, 15, 55
female, 15
cone biopsy, 26, 71, 81
congenital, 90
contagious, 90
contraception, 9, 14–17
after abortion, 86
barrier methods, 15–16
choosing a method, 14
hormonal methods,
16–17
intrauterine devices
(IUDs), 17
natural methods, 14–15
postcoital, 17, 68
contraceptives, 14, 15–17
counseling:
after abortion, 86
sexual, 49, 50, 61
culdoscopy, 84
cystitis, 25, 28–29, 32
cystocele, 30
cysts, 90
ovarian, 42–44

D

D&C (dilatation and
curettage), 82
see also cone biopsy, 81;
sterilization, 84; uterine
cancer, 45
depression, 34, 80
dermoid cysts, 42
DES, 26, 70, 71
diabetics, and thrush, 24
diaphragms, 15, 16
and cystitis, 29
and vaginal discharge,
23
diarrhea, 37, 40
diathermy, 40, 90
diuretics, 34, 90
drips, 90
dysmenorrhea, 10, 34, 37
dyspareunia, 46
dysplasia, 27, 71, 81

E

E. coli, 28
ectopic pregnancy, 68
  see also abnormal bleeding,
  36; chlamydia, 54; IUDs,
  17; menopause, 18
egg donation, 64
embryos, 8, 90
endometrial biopsy, 73
endometrial cancer, 45
endometriosis, 37, 40, 79
endometrium, 11
endoscopes, 90
enterocele, 30
ERPC (evacuation of the
  retained products of
  conception), 82
  see also miscarriage, 66,
  67; termination, 86
estrogen, 8, 10, 11
  lowered levels, 9

F, G

fallopian tubes, 9, 10
  blocked, 62, 63, 76
fear of penetration, 50
fertile period, 12–13
fertility:
  age and, 12
  and conception, 12–13
  cycle, 8–9
  end of, 9
  limiting, 9
  problems, 59–68
fertility medicines, 63
fertilization, 12
fibroids, 41, 78
  see also dysmenorrhea,
  37; menorrhagia, 38;
  miscarriage, 66
Flagyl, 25
fluid retention, 34
follicle-stimulating hormone
  (FSH), 11
functional cysts, 42
genital herpes, 52, 57
genital problems, 21–32
genital warts, 53, 71

gentian violet, 52
GIFT (gamete intra-fallopian
  transfer), 65
gonorrhea, 23, 54, 55

H

herbalism, 20
herpes, genital, 52, 57
HIV infection, 57–58
HMG (human menopausal
  gonadotropin), 63
homeopathy, 20
hormonal contraception, 16,
  17
hormone production, 10, 11
hormone replacement therapy,
  see HRT
hormones, 90
hot flushes, 9, 19
HPV (human papilloma virus),
  53
HRT (hormone replacement
  therapy), 9, 18, 19
  see also hysterectomy, 79;
  ovarian cysts, 43; pruritis
  vulvae, 22
HSG (hysterosalpingogram),
  67, 76
hysterectomy, 18, 79–80
  avoiding, 74, 78
  radical, 27, 79
  see also amenorrhea, 35;
  endometrial biopsy, 73;
  fibroids, 41;
  menorrhagia, 38; PID,
  46; prolapse, 30;
  sterilization, 83; uterine
  cancer, 45
hysterosalpingogram (HSG),
  67, 76
hysteroscopy, 38, 41, 74, 82
hysterotomy, 86

I

ICSI (intracytoplasmic sperm
  injection), 65
idoxuridine, 52
immune system, 57, 90

implants, contraceptive, 16
in vitro fertilization (IVF), 40,
  63, 64–65
incontinence, 32
induced labor termination,
  86
induced termination, 67, 85
infectious diseases, 90
infertility, 60–65
  assisted conception, 63–65
  female problems, 60–61
  male problems, 60
  shared problems, 61
  testing for, 62
  treatment, 62–63
  see also endometriosis,
  40; PID, 46
insomnia,19
instant menopause, 79
intercourse, sexual:
  after abortion, 86
  after miscarriage, 67
  after vaginal sterilization,
  84
  bleeding after, 36
  during menstruation, 11
  frequent, 13, 29
  painful, 48
  see also chlamydia, 54;
  endometriosis, 40;
  fibroids, 41; ovarian
  cysts, 42; PID, 46;
  prolapse, 30, 31; thrush,
  24; vaginismus, 50
intrauterine devices
  see IUDs
iron-rich foods, 38
itchiness of the vulva, 22, 23
IUDs (intrauterine devices),
  14, 17
  and breakthrough
  bleeding, 36
  and ectopic pregnancy, 17,
  68
  and gonorrhea, 55
  and heavy periods, 38
  and PID, 17, 46
  and vaginal discharge, 23
IVF (in vitro fertilization), 40,
  63, 64–65

J, K, L

Kegel exercises, 30, 31, 32
keratin, 90
laparoscopes, 90
laparoscopy, 77
  see also ectopic pregnancy,
    68; endometriosis, 40;
    fertility problems, 62;
    fibroids, 41; HSG, 76;
    ovarian cysts, 42; PID,
    46; sterilization, 84
laparotomy, 84
LAVH (laparoscopic assisted
  vaginal hysterectomy), 80
LLETZ (large loop excision of
  the transformation zone),
  26, 72, 81
LH (luteinizing hormone)
  predictor kits, 64
low-dose mini-pills, 14, 16, 68
lymph, 91

M

mammography, 91
marriage guidance clinics, 50
menarche,10, 91
menopause, 9, 18–20
  bleeding during, 36
  instant, 79
  natural remedies, 20
  predicting, 18
  seeing the doctor, 19–20
  self-help, 20
  stages, 18
  symptoms, 9, 19
menorrhagia, 36, 38, 82
menstrual cycle, 10, 11
menstrual hygiene, 11
menstrual problems, 10,
  33–38, 40
menstruation, 9, 10–11
  abnormal bleeding, 36;
  heavy *see* endometriosis,
    40; fibroids, 41;
    menorrhagia, 38;
    ovarian cysts, 42;
    uterine cancer, 45
  interrupted, 35
  starting late, 35
metronidazole drugs, 25

mini-pills, 14, 16, 68
miscarriage, 36, 66–67
mood changes, 34
mucus method, 13
myomectomy, 41, 78

N, O

Neisseria gonorrhoeae, 55
night sweats, 9, 19
nipples:
  changes during pregnancy, 9
  sore, 10
nonspecific urethritis, 54
oral thrush, 24, 57
ovarian cancer, 18, 44
ovarian cysts, 42–44
  and IUDs, 17
ovaries, 10
  in embryo, 8
ovulation, 10, 12
  home test kits, 14
oxytocin, 86

P

Pap smear, 71
pedicle, twisted, 42
pelvic examination, 42, 70
pelvic floor muscles, 31, 32
pelvic inflammatory disease
  (PID), 46
  and IUDs, 17, 46
  see also chlamydia, 54;
    ectopic pregnancy, 68;
    gonorrhea, 55
pelvic problems, 39–46
pelvic soreness, 37
penetration, fear of, 50
penicillin, 54, 55, 56
perimenopause, 18
perineum, sore, 25, 55
periods (menstrual):
  bleeding between, 36, 45
  cessation of, 8, 18, 35
  heavy *see* endometriosis
    40; fibroids, 41;
    menorrhagia, 38;
    ovarian cysts, 42;
periods *continued*
    uterine cancer, 45
    painful, 37, 42

pessaries, 91
Pfannenstiel incisions, 78
PID *see* pelvic inflammatory
  disease
pills, contraceptive, 14, 16
  and breakthrough
    bleeding, 37
  for relief of dysmenorrhea,
    37
  see also ovarian cancer, 44;
    thrush, 24
pituitary gland, 11
placental insufficiency, 66
PMS (premenstrual
  syndrome), 10, 34
pneumonia, 57
podophyllin,53
polycystic ovarian syndrome,
  43
polyps, 23, 91
postcoital contraception, 17,
  68
posterior repair, 30
postmenopausal bleeding, 45
postmenopause, 18
pregnancy, 9
  bleeding during, 36
  early symptoms, 12
  ectopic, 68
  multiple, 63
  preventing *see* contraception
  termination, 85–86
  tubal, 68
  ultrasound scanning, 75
premenopause, 10, 12, 18
premenstrual syndrome
  (PMS), 10, 34
progesterone, 8, 10, 11
progesterone blood tests, 62
progesterone IUDs, 14, 17
  and dysmenorrhea, 37
  and menorrhagia, 38
progesterone-only pill, 14, 16,
  68
progesterone therapy 34
prolapse, 30–31, 79, 80
  and urinary problems, 28,
  32
prostaglandin, 34, 37
  and termination, 85
providone iodine solution,
  52

pruritis vulvae, 22
puberty, 8
  late development, 35
pus, 91

R, S

radiation therapy, 27, 91
rectal prolapse, 30
rectocele, 30
reproductive organs, 10
salpingostomy, 63
sarcoma, 91
secondary, 91
sex, determined by genes, 12
sex drive, lack of, 19, 48, 49
sexual counseling, 49, 50, 61
sexual intercourse *see*
  intercourse, sexual
sexual problems, 47–50
sexually transmitted diseases,
  11, 51–58
shingles, 57
smear tests, 26, 27, 52, 71
speculum examination, 70
sperm:
  donation of, 64
  survival period, 12
spermicides, 16
sponges, contraceptive, 15, 16
sterilization, 83–84
  hysterectomy as, 79
  male, 83, 84
stress incontinence, 30, 31, 32
subfertility, 46, 61
suction termination, 85–86
sweating, 9, 19
symptothermal method, 14
syphilis, 56

T

tampons, 11, 23, 29
temperature method, for
  predicting fertile period, 13
termination of pregnancy,
  85–86
test tube babies *see* in vitro
  fertilization
testosterone, 49
tetracyclines, 29, 54
throat, sore, 55

thrush, 22, 23, 24
thyroid gland, underactive, 49
tissue, 91
trachylectomy, 27
Treponema pallidum, 56
trichloroacetic acid, 53
trichomoniasis, 23, 25
tubal ligation, 77, 83, 84
tubal pregnancy, 68
tuberculosis, 46

U, V

ulcer, 91
ultrasound scan, 75
  see also ectopic pregnancy,
    68; endometrial biopsy,
    73; fertility problems,
    62; fibroids, 41;
    miscarriage, 66; ovarian
    cysts, 42, 43
urethrocele, 30
urethral prolapse, 30
urinary antiseptics, 29
urination:
  frequent *see* cystitis, 28;
    dysmenorrhea, 37;
    ovarian cancer, 44;
    prolapse, 30; uterine
    cancer, 45
  painful *see* cystitis 28;
    genital herpes, 52;
    pruritis vulvae, 22;
    trichomoniasis, 25
  problems *see* fibroids, 41;
    ovarian cysts, 42
urine:
  alkalinizing, 29
  discolored, 28
  involuntary leakage, 31–32
uterine cancer, 18, 41, 45
uterine prolapse, 30, 80
uterus, 10
  changes in pregnancy, 9
  removal of, 79–80
  ultrasound scan, 73, 75
vagina, 10
  involuntary closing, 50
vaginal deodorants, 24
vaginal discharge, 10, 23
vaginal dryness, 9, 19, 48
vaginal hysterectomy, 80

vaginal itching, 25
vaginal spotting of blood, 36,
  46, 66
vaginal sterilization, 84
vaginal thrush, 24
vaginismus, 48, 50
vasectomy, 83, 84
venereal, 91
vulva, itchiness of, 22, 23

W, X

warts, genital, 53, 71, 91
withdrawal method, 15
X rays, 76, 91

ACKNOWLEDGMENTS

The publisher would like to thank the following individuals and organizations for their contribution to this book.

ILLUSTRATION
Dave Ashby, Joanna Cameron, Tony Graham, Aziz Khan, John Lang, Joe Lawrence, Andrew Macdonald, Kevin Marks, Annabel Milne, Coral Mula, Sheilagh Noble, Howard Pemberton, Jim Robins, Sue Smith, Sue Sharples, Emma Whiting, Paul Williams, Lydia Umney

MEDICAL CONSULTANTS
Samir A. Alvi MB,
Elizabeth Owen MD

ADDITIONAL EDITORIAL ASSISTANCE
Nicky Adamson, Claire Cross, Maureen Rissik
Constance M. Robinson

EQUIPMENT
Boots The Chemist, Marie Stopes Health Clinics

TEXT FILM
The Brightside Partnership, London